# A Castor Oil Healing Book

CRAFTED BY SKRIUWER

Copyright © 2024 by Skriuwer.

All rights reserved. No part of this book may be used or reproduced in any form whatsoever without written permission except in the case of brief quotations in critical articles or reviews.

For more information, contact : **kontakt@skriuwer.com** (www.skriuwer.com)

# TABLE OF CONTENTS

## CHAPTER 1: INTRODUCTION TO CASTOR OIL

- History of the castor plant and its seeds
- Main properties and traits of castor oil
- Overview of common uses and reasons people turn to it

## CHAPTER 2: HISTORY AND EARLY USE

- Role of castor oil in ancient cultures
- Spread of castor oil through trade routes
- Traditional practices in folk medicine

## CHAPTER 3: CHEMICAL STRUCTURE AND KEY PARTS

- Breakdown of fatty acids, especially ricinoleic acid
- Explanation of thickness and distinct properties
- Why castor oil differs from other plant oils

## CHAPTER 4: HARVESTING AND PROCESSING

- How castor seeds are grown and collected
- Methods of extracting the oil
- Quality control and refining steps

## CHAPTER 5: HEALTHY SKIN SUPPORT

- Benefits of castor oil for dryness and rough patches
- Ways to apply castor oil to keep skin soft
- Combining castor oil with light oils for daily routines

## CHAPTER 6: HAIR AND SCALP CARE

- How castor oil can reduce hair dryness
- Pre-shampoo treatments and scalp massages
- Mixing castor oil with other ingredients for hair masks

## CHAPTER 7: DIGESTIVE SUPPORT

- Castor oil's role as a laxative
- Safe dosing guidelines and precautions
- Considering alternatives and when to seek help

## CHAPTER 8: IMMUNE SYSTEM EFFECTS

- Possible mild support through castor oil packs
- Role of relaxation and decreased stress
- Why research on immune benefits is still emerging

## CHAPTER 9: LIVER AND ORGAN HEALTH

- Traditional belief in applying castor oil packs over the liver
- Steps to do it safely and watch for changes
- Balancing castor oil use with healthy lifestyle habits

## CHAPTER 10: STRESS AND SLEEP SUPPORT

- Castor oil foot rubs, packs, and gentle massages
- Nighttime routines for relaxation
- Tips on combining castor oil with calming habits

## CHAPTER 11: JOINT AND MUSCLE RELIEF

- Ways castor oil might soothe mild aches
- Using packs or rubs on knees, shoulders, and other spots
- Blending with heat for extra comfort

## CHAPTER 12: HORMONE BALANCE

- Castor oil's possible role in supporting normal hormone function
- Applying warm packs over lower abdomen or liver area
- Importance of diet and stress management in overall balance

## CHAPTER 13: HOME REMEDIES FOR PARENTS AND CHILDREN

- Safety rules for using castor oil around kids
- Small remedies for dry skin, hair tangles, and mild tummy complaints
- Avoiding oral use for young children unless guided by a professional

## CHAPTER 14: PET AND ANIMAL USES

- Limited, careful external application on paws or minor dry patches
- Warnings about cat sensitivities and licking
- When to seek a vet's input

## CHAPTER 15: EXTERNAL THERAPIES

- Step-by-step for castor oil packs
- Tips for adding gentle heat
- Rub and massage routines for quick daily use

## CHAPTER 16: SAFETY MEASURES & WARNINGS

- Identifying allergic reactions and safe storage
- Guidelines for internal consumption and age-related cautions
- Properly handling and storing castor oil to avoid rancidity

## CHAPTER 17: MIXING WITH OTHER OILS & HERBS

- Reasons to blend castor oil for lighter texture
- Common mix recipes for skin, hair, and massage
- Infusing castor oil with herbs or essential oils

# CHAPTER 18: MODERN RESEARCH AND STUDIES

- *Overview of scientific findings on castor oil*
- *Focus on ricinoleic acid and potential benefits*
- *Gaps in current research and future directions*

# CHAPTER 19: REAL-LIFE STORIES AND HELPFUL EXAMPLES

- *Everyday scenarios where castor oil fits into routines*
- *Parents, athletes, students, and hobbyists sharing their tips*
- *Practical lessons from real-life experiences*

# CHAPTER 20: COMMON QUESTIONS AND FINAL THOUGHTS

- *Frequently asked questions about castor oil use*
- *Advice on choosing products and maintaining routines*
- *Wrap-up of key points and encouragement for safe experimentation*

# CHAPTER 1: INTRODUCTION TO CASTOR OIL

Castor oil is a thick plant-based oil that comes from the seeds of the castor plant. The castor plant is known by the scientific name *Ricinus communis*. These seeds contain a substance that can be harmful if not processed correctly. However, when people press the seeds to get the oil, the harmful parts are removed, leaving a thick liquid that has been used for many purposes.

Castor oil has been part of home remedies for many years. It has a texture that stands out among plant oils. Many other plant oils feel lighter or have a different smell, but castor oil is known for its thickness. This thickness is connected to the high amount of a special fat called ricinoleic acid. Ricinoleic acid is not often found in large amounts in most other oils that come from plants. That is one key reason castor oil can be so useful for personal care and other basic uses.

## General Idea of Castor Oil

Castor oil often appears pale yellow or slightly clear. Some types might look a bit greenish or brownish, depending on how they are pressed and filtered. The smell of castor oil can be mild or somewhat strong. Many people notice that it feels sticky compared to lighter oils like almond oil or olive oil. This quality can make it stand out when you use it on your skin or hair.

Although some people might find the texture of castor oil to be heavy, that same thickness can be helpful. When you rub it on your skin, it may hold moisture better than lighter oils. When used on the scalp and hair, it can coat each strand, making hair feel smooth and possibly look shiny. Over time, many have found that a small amount of castor oil can give their hair a healthy look. Others apply a small dab to patches of dry skin.

It is helpful to know that castor oil is not just something you can rub on your skin or hair. It has also been used in small amounts for the digestive system. However, care is needed here. Swallowing too much castor oil can cause strong bowel effects, such as cramping or a sudden need to find a bathroom. For a long time, some people used castor oil to help with constipation. But you must be careful about how much you use, because an overdose can lead to discomfort.

---

## Basic Science Behind Castor Oil

A big reason castor oil is special is because of the large amount of ricinoleic acid. This is a type of fatty acid. Fatty acids are the basic building blocks in fats and oils. Many plant oils have more common fats such as oleic acid or linoleic acid. Castor oil does have some of these, but it is the ricinoleic acid that gives it certain properties different from most other oils.

Ricinoleic acid is sometimes linked to calming properties when rubbed on the skin. Some research suggests that applying castor oil to skin areas that are dry or rough could help the skin stay soft. Some people also say that the ricinoleic acid helps reduce minor swelling or redness when used over time. This effect might explain why some individuals find it soothing to use castor oil packs on sore areas of the body.

When people discuss castor oil, they often bring up the words "castor oil pack." This is a piece of cloth that has been soaked in warm castor oil. The cloth is placed on the body, usually the abdomen or an area that needs comfort. Some then cover it with plastic wrap or another layer to keep in the warmth and prevent mess. People may use a heating pad or hot water bottle to keep it warm for a while. This method allows the oil to rest on the skin for an extended period. However, there are steps and safety measures to keep in mind, such as checking the skin to make sure there is no reaction.

## Variety in Types of Castor Oil

There is not just one type of castor oil on the market. Some castor oils are labeled as "cold-pressed," meaning they are extracted without using high heat. This method is said to keep more of the natural parts of the oil in place. Other castor oils might be refined through heat or chemical methods. Some consumers prefer cold-pressed castor oil because they believe it is closer to its natural state.

Another type is "black castor oil," often known as Jamaican black castor oil. This type is made by roasting or heating the castor seeds before pressing them. This process gives the oil a darker color and a different smell. Some believe Jamaican black castor oil is extra strong for hair care, but this can come down to personal preference. Many find that any high-quality castor oil can work if used correctly.

---

## Where Castor Oil Comes From

The castor plant can grow in many places around the world, though it is found mostly in tropical or subtropical regions. It can grow quite tall under the right conditions. The seeds grow inside pods that appear on the plant. Once harvested, these seeds are processed to remove the oil. Because the seeds contain ricin, a toxic substance, they must be handled with care. Manufacturers make sure the final product is free from harmful parts.

Not everyone realizes that although raw castor seeds can be harmful, the oil is safe when produced by correct methods. This is a key fact that shows how careful processes can turn a possibly harmful seed into a helpful product. Through pressing, filtering, and sometimes other steps, the castor oil is separated from parts that can cause harm. That is why it is important to buy castor oil from a trusted source.

## Common Uses and Observations

People use castor oil for many reasons at home. Some rub it on their elbows, knees, or feet to make them feel less rough. Others might blend a little castor oil with lighter oils, such as jojoba or grape seed oil, to make it easier to apply on larger parts of the skin. Since castor oil is thick, mixing it can help spread it more evenly. Some also mix castor oil with certain essential oils, though care is needed to avoid skin irritation.

The appearance of the hair can sometimes improve with castor oil use. People who have hair that tends to be dry or that breaks easily might find that a small amount of castor oil helps protect the strands. They sometimes rub a bit into their scalp as well. The scalp can get itchy or dry, and castor oil might help with that. But it is wise to start with a small amount, because too much can weigh the hair down or make it look oily.

In addition, some older home tips recommend castor oil for mild eye-related needs, like an ingredient in homemade lip and eyelash treatments. However, one should be extra careful when applying anything near the eyes. Some people might talk about dropping castor oil in their eyes, but this is risky without professional guidance. Products labeled for cosmetic or external use might not be purified enough for the eyes. So always look at the label and ask a trained health person before using castor oil in the eyes.

---

## Overview of Internal Use

While castor oil has a long list of external uses, it also has been used internally in certain cases. A small measured amount might help with constipation. It works by triggering the bowels to move. But if you take too much, it can cause cramps, diarrhea, or dehydration. Pregnant people have sometimes been told about castor oil to support contractions, but this is something to be done only under professional supervision. Using castor oil this way might be uncomfortable and is not something to do without guidance.

For most users, taking castor oil by mouth is less common than using it externally. The taste can also be quite strong and unpleasant to some people. If you do plan to take it by mouth, you must check guidelines from a reliable source or a health worker. Knowing the right dose and timing is key. More is not always better, since it can stress the body.

## Comparing Castor Oil with Other Oils

It can be helpful to compare castor oil to better-known oils. For instance, coconut oil is also used for hair and skin. Coconut oil tends to be solid at cooler temperatures and melts at body temperature. Castor oil, on the other hand, stays a thick liquid even when it is quite cold. Olive oil is widely used in cooking, but it is not as sticky. Olive oil also has a gentler smell and feel compared to castor oil.

People might ask why they should pick castor oil over these other oils. Castor oil's main draw is its unique fatty acid profile, especially the ricinoleic acid. It can hold moisture in a way that some other oils might not. Some also feel that castor oil can soothe the skin more effectively in certain areas, like cracked heels or thick skin on the soles of the feet. However, every person has different needs, so some might prefer lighter oils.

## Factors to Consider Before Using Castor Oil

1. **Allergy or Sensitivity:** A small number of people might have a sensitivity to castor oil. It is always smart to do a test on a small patch of skin first. Apply a tiny drop of castor oil on your forearm and wait a day to see if there is any redness or itching. If there is none, you are likely safe to use it in larger areas.
2. **Purity:** Look for castor oil that says "cold-pressed" or "100% pure" if you want a product that has not been combined with other ingredients. This can help avoid extra chemicals that might irritate your skin.

3. **Storage:** Castor oil does not have to be refrigerated. Keep it in a cool, dark place if possible. Try to keep the lid sealed to prevent contamination.
4. **Interaction with Medicines:** If you plan to swallow castor oil, check with a health professional. It could interact with some medicines or health conditions. For external use, interactions are less common.
5. **Ethical and Environmental Aspects:** Some people want to know how the castor plants are grown and harvested. Organic castor oil might be available, and some brands share details about how they support farmers.

## Myths and Facts

Because castor oil has been around so long, there are a number of myths about its uses. One myth is that castor oil can cure all kinds of serious diseases if you just rub it on your body. There is no strong evidence to back up such claims. Another myth is that castor oil is deadly if you put it on your skin. That confusion might come from the fact that raw castor seeds are dangerous due to ricin. The oil, however, is considered safe when it is properly made.

A fact about castor oil is that it can help keep moisture in the skin, because it reduces water loss. Another fact is that it can help the bowels move if taken by mouth, but only if done with care. Some people think castor oil is the single best hair growth solution. While many share positive stories about hair thickness after using castor oil, more formal research is still needed. It may be that the oil helps reduce dryness and breakage, so hair looks and feels healthier, rather than directly causing faster hair growth.

## Possible Future Uses

Researchers are still studying castor oil for new and better ways to apply it. Because ricinoleic acid can fight certain germs in lab tests, there might be uses in creams or lotions that help with minor skin problems. Some scientists are looking at ways castor oil could be part of packaging materials to keep items fresh. The thickness and protective qualities could have uses in manufacturing. Others wonder if castor oil could play a bigger role in biodegradable products, since it comes from a plant source and breaks down more easily than synthetic materials.

## Avoiding Overuse

One important point about castor oil is that you should avoid overuse, especially when swallowing it. While it might help with constipation from time to time, using it every day can lead to problems. Your digestive system can become too dependent on it, or you could develop nutritional problems due to your body moving food too quickly. Moderation is key with any strong remedy.

For external use, people often find they do not need large amounts. Because castor oil is thick, a little can go a long way. If you use too much on your scalp or hair, it might take a lot of shampoo to wash it out. It might also attract dust or lint if you do not rinse or wipe away the excess. So use only as much as you need, and pay attention to how your skin or hair reacts over time.

## Helpful Tips for Beginners

- **Start Slowly:** If you are new to castor oil, try it on a small patch of skin before using larger amounts.
- **Mix It:** If you find castor oil too thick for your liking, blend it with another light oil in a small bowl. You could use equal parts of castor oil and a light oil like argan oil. Then rub this blend into your skin or hair.
- **Warm It Gently:** For external use, some people like to warm the oil slightly by placing a small bottle of castor oil into a bowl of warm water. This makes it easier to apply.
- **Use Soft Cloth:** If you plan to do a castor oil pack, use a soft cotton cloth or flannel. Place the oil-soaked cloth on your skin and cover

with plastic wrap. Then place a heating pad or hot water bottle on top. Watch that it does not get too hot and cause burns.
- **Time Limit:** Some people leave a castor oil pack on for 30 minutes, while others leave it for up to an hour. You can test different times to see what feels best.
- **Wash Off:** After using castor oil on your skin, wash or wipe off any excess. This can help avoid stains on clothes or bedding.

---

## Special Points That May Not Be Widely Known

1. **Reaction to Light:** Castor oil can become cloudy or change color if it is exposed to sunlight for a long time. Some suggest storing it in dark or amber-colored bottles to help keep it stable.
2. **Use in Massaging the Gums:** Some individuals rub a tiny amount of high-quality castor oil on their gums. They claim that it helps keep their gums feeling soft. However, it is best to be sure that you use an oil labeled safe for oral use.
3. **Gentle on Eyebrows and Eyelashes:** Some people lightly apply castor oil to their eyebrows or eyelashes to make them look thicker. If you do this, be sure not to get any oil in your eyes. Use a clean spoolie brush or a cotton swab.
4. **Industrial Use:** Besides personal care, castor oil is also used in industries like lubricants, paints, and more. The same unique fatty acid structure that helps your skin can also help machines run smoothly.
5. **In Soaps and Balms:** Castor oil is a popular ingredient in homemade soaps. It can help create a rich lather. Some lip balms also use castor oil because it helps keep lips soft.

---

## Recognizing Quality

When picking a castor oil product, look at the label to see if it lists where the oil was made. Some manufacturers provide details about how the seeds are grown. If you are interested in organic options, you can look for a certification seal. If you are not worried about organic status, you can still check for any signs of added ingredients or fragrances that might cause irritation.

Another way to test the quality is to feel and smell the oil. A pure cold-pressed castor oil usually has a mild scent. If you notice a very strong or foul smell, it might be old or contaminated. Also, the oil should be mostly clear or pale yellow if it is refined. Jamaican black castor oil will have a darker hue, but it should not look cloudy or chunky. Any sign of mold or foreign bits could mean it is not safe to use.

## Simple Ways to Include Castor Oil in Daily Life

- **Lotion Booster:** Add a few drops of castor oil to your usual lotion. Mix it in your hands before you apply it to your body. This might make the lotion feel richer.
- **Foot Soak Add-In:** Some people put a small amount of castor oil into their foot soak water. It might help soften rough spots.
- **Cuticle Care:** After washing your hands, rub a drop of castor oil into each cuticle. Do this for a few days to see if you notice a difference.
- **Frizz Tamer:** If you have frizzy hair, rub a tiny bit of castor oil (mixed with a lighter oil if you wish) between your hands, then gently pat down any stray hairs.
- **Bath Time Treatment:** You could put a tablespoon of castor oil in your bath water. Be cautious, though, as it can make the tub slippery. This may help keep your skin from feeling too dry after a bath.

## Possible Questions You Might Have

1. **Why is castor oil sometimes linked to negative outcomes in history?**
   In some places, people were forced to drink castor oil as a form of punishment or intimidation. This past misuse led to a negative view of the oil for some time. However, when used wisely for health reasons, it can be helpful.

2. **Do I have to buy a special brand for hair or skin, or can I use any food-grade castor oil?**
   Often, any high-quality oil can be used on the body. Food-grade castor oil might be safe, but it is still wise to confirm it is labeled for external use as well. Different brands might refine their oil in different ways, so check for any mention on the label about external vs. internal use.
3. **Is castor oil safe for children?**
   Many parents use castor oil for their children in small amounts, like on dry skin. But always talk to a health professional before giving castor oil by mouth to a child. Children's bodies are more sensitive, and dosages need to be correct.
4. **Can I grow my own castor plant?**
   Castor plants can be grown in home gardens, but they might need a warm climate. Remember that the seeds are toxic if eaten raw. If you plan to harvest them, you must learn the proper steps for safety.
5. **Will it stain my clothes?**
   Castor oil can leave oil spots that might be tough to remove. If you are using castor oil on your skin, wear older clothes until you see if the oil rubs off. Use towels that you do not mind getting stained if you are doing a castor oil pack.

# CHAPTER 2: HISTORY AND EARLY USE

Castor oil has a long record of use that stretches across many parts of the world. It has been mentioned in old texts, found in Egyptian tombs, and recognized as a part of health practices in far-off places. To fully appreciate how castor oil became part of daily life for so many people, it helps to look at how ancient cultures first discovered the castor plant, learned to press the oil from its seeds, and found uses for the thick liquid.

In this chapter, we will review some of the oldest known facts about castor oil and how these facts shaped its role in different societies. We will talk about how early people pressed the seeds, how they tested the oil for safety, and the many ways they thought it could help the body. By the end, you will have a deeper picture of how castor oil started its path into modern health routines.

## Castor Oil in Ancient Times

One of the earliest places where castor oil is noted is in ancient Egypt. Historical records suggest that Egyptians used castor oil for lamps. Because the oil can burn steadily, it was an option for lighting before electricity. Imagine trying to read or work in an old Egyptian home late at night; lamps fueled with castor oil might have been a solution to keep the room lit. Some accounts also propose that ancient Egyptians used castor oil on their skin and hair, as personal appearance was important in that culture. Scenes on walls and writings hint that smooth skin and healthy hair were signs of good living, and castor oil may have been one of the items used for these goals.

Egyptians were also known for their beauty preparations. They used oils, creams, and salves made from a variety of substances. Castor oil's thick nature might have been useful for mixing with other ingredients. They might have combined castor oil with fragrant plants or other oils to create a spreadable lotion or ointment. While there are not many precise recipes that have survived in detail, references to "castor seeds" or "oil from castor seeds" appear in some ancient documents, indicating that it held a place in the list of common items.

Another area of early mention is the region that is now India. Some writings suggest that the castor plant grew there and was cultivated for its seeds. People may have used castor oil in small amounts as a purgative—something that helped them rid the body of waste. This was done carefully, since even small amounts can have a strong effect on the bowels. Others might have used it for lamp oil as well. Over time, knowledge of this oil likely spread through trade and communication between different regions, making castor oil known across various cultural groups.

## Spread to Other Cultures

As people traveled, traded goods, and shared ideas, castor oil began to appear in many other places. Ancient Greek and Roman writers mention it in some of their works. They also talk about the castor plant, noting its strange seed pods and how they contained an oil that was quite potent. Some healers of the time may have recommended castor oil for certain ailments, though the records are scattered.

Over centuries, castor oil made its way into Persia (now Iran), into parts of Africa beyond Egypt, and even into China. Each place found its own ways to use the oil. In some cultures, it became a base for traditional medicines. People might have combined it with herbs or minerals to create pastes for the skin. In others, it was considered mostly good as lamp oil, since it burned with a consistent flame. This wide range of uses shows how flexible castor oil was, even in times when technology was simple.

It is important to note that in many of these early uses, people had to be careful about the raw seeds. Some societies found that if you ate the seed without removing the toxic parts, it could be deadly. This knowledge was likely passed down in families or through local healers. Over time, they discovered pressing methods or ways of cooking that allowed them to separate the oil from the harmful proteins in the seed. Through these steps, they could get a safer product.

## Historical Pressing Methods

How did ancient people get the oil out of castor seeds before modern machines existed? They used various simple devices or methods. One common way was to crush the seeds between stones. Another method was to grind them in a mortar and pestle, then wrap the ground seeds in cloth and press them to squeeze out the oil. The leftover seed cake could be used for certain purposes, though it is not edible. In some places, they might have heated the crushed seeds to make the oil flow more easily.

Of course, these methods were not as refined as modern ones, so the oil might have been darker and contained bits of seed or other impurities. People might have let the oil sit in a container so that heavier particles settled at the bottom, making it easier to skim off the clearer oil on top. Such steps probably varied from region to region. As time went on, better tools were invented, making it simpler to extract more oil in less time.

Because the pressing process in older times required physical labor, castor oil might have been seen as a valuable product. Not everyone had the knowledge or the tools to do it well, so there may have been special tradespeople who sold castor oil to those who needed it. This trade contributed to the spread of the oil, as people traveling from one place to another might carry it to sell or barter.

## Role in Folk Medicine

Throughout history, individuals in different cultures found uses for castor oil in folk medicine. For example, some might have rubbed it on the stomach to help with certain ailments. Others might have used warm compresses of castor oil on aching joints or tight muscles. Because of its thick quality, castor oil could stay on the skin for a long time, which might have enhanced its soothing properties.

In places with strong herbal traditions, castor oil might have been an ingredient in salves or ointments. These mixtures might include ground herbs, beeswax, and castor oil. The final product could be stored in small containers for use on rashes or insect bites. Although we do not have detailed scientific records from every culture, we have enough bits of information that show castor oil was recognized for its potential benefits.

Some societies also used castor oil on animals. For example, if livestock had certain skin issues, people might apply castor oil to the affected area. It could help keep the area moist and guard it against some types of pests. This kind of practice likely came from observing that castor oil was thick enough to create a protective layer.

## Early Trade and Value

The trade of castor oil has a long past. Because it could be used for lamps, for personal care, and in certain old medicines, it was a product of interest. Merchants carried it along trade routes, sometimes in clay jars or animal skins. In some eras, it might have been sold at markets alongside other oils such as olive oil or sesame oil. Each oil had different properties, so people bought them for different reasons.

Over time, as shipping improved, castor oil could be moved more quickly from one region to another. Eventually, when ships began to cross oceans, castor oil from areas where the castor plant grew well could be exported to places where it did not grow. In this way, castor oil gained a broader audience. People in colder climates learned about it, and it began to appear in their folk remedies as well. Some documents show that by the 18th and 19th centuries, castor oil was known across Europe and parts of North America as both a health aid and an industrial ingredient.

## Influence of Key Historical Figures

Some historical figures, such as early medical practitioners, might have written about castor oil's effects. For example, a Greek physician might have noted how castor oil was used to clear the bowels, while an Egyptian scribe might have recorded how it was applied to the scalp. These writings, though not always detailed, helped build the knowledge that was passed on through the ages.

In the 19th century, as modern medicine started to take shape, doctors began to analyze castor oil's uses more scientifically. It became a product that pharmacies stocked, often labeled as a laxative. Doctors and pharmacists might have recommended it for constipation or for certain skin problems. However, as more synthetic products came on the market in the 20th century, castor oil's role in mainstream medicine shifted. Despite that shift, many families still kept a bottle at home.

One negative historical episode involved the misuse of castor oil in some political contexts, where it was forced on people as a form of punishment or humiliation. This caused some to associate castor oil with negative feelings. However, outside of these forced uses, many still recognized its health benefits.

---

## Castor Oil in Early American Life

When European settlers arrived in the Americas, they brought with them some knowledge of castor oil, though the plant might have also existed in certain tropical parts of the Americas. By the 18th and 19th centuries, castor oil was sometimes grown and pressed locally. Historical records show that people used it much the same way they did in other parts of the world. It was a remedy for constipation, a base for salves, and a possible lamp fuel.

Families might have passed down their own methods for using castor oil. For instance, a grandmother might teach her children how to apply a warm castor oil pack on the abdomen to soothe aches. A father might keep a small tin of castor oil in the barn to apply to farm animals' minor wounds. These family practices were part of everyday life in many rural areas. Some older diaries and letters even talk about the unpleasant taste of castor oil when used for digestive help, showing it was well known for that purpose.

## Early Research Observations

Even before modern science could break down the exact structure of fats in castor oil, observers made some informal notes on its properties. They noticed that when the oil sat in a container for a while, it did not become rancid as fast as certain other oils. They also found that it did not freeze in cold weather as easily as some other plant oils. These traits made it useful for different tasks. For example, it might have been used to lubricate small machinery parts long before big factories appeared.

Some old texts also mention that castor oil could be used on the eyes of animals like horses, to keep them clear of certain pests or to soothe irritation. This may not be recommended today without professional guidance, but it shows that people looked at castor oil as something that might protect and soothe. Over time, these kinds of observations built up a body of knowledge, so that by the time modern scientists began to study castor oil, they already had a backlog of folk ideas to test.

## Religious and Cultural Practices

In some cultural or religious groups, oils played a part in certain ceremonies or rites. Castor oil, being accessible in certain regions, might have been used in lamps for places of worship. The steady flame from castor oil could have made it suitable for temples or shrines that needed continuous light. Some might have also used it on the skin as a sign of purification or anointment, mixing it with scents or herbs. The details can vary widely between groups, but it highlights how oils could hold a spiritual or symbolic meaning as well.

## Shift to Modern Times

As centuries passed, better methods of processing changed how castor oil was produced. In the late 19th and early 20th century, mechanical presses and eventually hydraulic or screw presses allowed manufacturers to produce castor oil in greater volumes with better consistency. Then came chemical processes that could refine the oil to remove strong odors or colors.

With industrialization, castor oil found more roles. It was used in making soaps, lubricants, and even some types of plastics. Scientists discovered that the thick nature of castor oil and its special fats could help create materials with certain flexible properties. This industrial demand led to large-scale farms dedicated to growing castor plants. However, this also meant that castor oil became a commodity, subject to market changes and global trade patterns.

On the personal care side, pharmaceutical companies started to package castor oil in bottles with labels indicating dosage and uses. By the mid-20th century, many drugstores sold castor oil as a household remedy. Mothers who remembered receiving a spoonful of castor oil as children might have done the same for their own children, passing down the practice. However, the taste was often dreaded, leading some children to hide when they saw the castor oil bottle come out.

---

## Traditional vs. Scientific Views

Though castor oil had been used in folk medicine for ages, modern science took time to explore how it worked. Early on, there was some doubt among doctors and scientists as to whether castor oil really had all the benefits people claimed. Over the 19th and 20th centuries, more formal lab research began to identify ricinoleic acid and how it affected the body. Tests in animals and eventually humans showed that castor oil does indeed stimulate the bowel to contract, explaining why it worked as a laxative.

At the same time, scientists looked at whether it could help skin conditions. Lab studies on skin cells and small clinical trials hinted that castor oil might soothe certain types of irritation. Researchers also found some evidence that it might help with fungal growth on the skin. However, these studies varied in size and scope. The knowledge was not as detailed or widespread as some might hope. Still, the blend of folk wisdom and emerging science helped keep castor oil in the public eye.

## Historical Lessons for Today

Why does the history of castor oil matter? It shows how people observed the natural world, tested different plants, and found uses that fit their needs. They learned to press seeds, to remove harmful parts, and to store the oil. They passed on tips for using it for lamps, cooking, or personal care. These methods laid the groundwork for the modern usage of castor oil.

From ancient lamps in Egypt to family remedies in rural America, castor oil has touched many lives. It has been part of trade, medicine, and industry. Understanding this past might help us see why castor oil remains popular in certain circles. Even though we now have synthetic products and advanced medicines, there is still value in this old oil. People continue to experiment with it, coming up with new ways to apply it or mix it with other items.

## Modern Recognition of Ancient Practices

Today, some companies market castor oil in ways that tie back to its long heritage. They may label products as "ancient formula" or "traditional method." While the marketing might be catchy, it does point to the fact that castor oil's use is nothing new. It has stood the test of time, in a sense. If it had not offered something useful, it might have faded from memory long ago.

On the flip side, we have learned from history that not all uses were safe or kind. Forced consumption of castor oil as punishment is a sad chapter. The toxic seeds reminded people that nature has dangers. But the good news is that much of this knowledge—both the positive and negative—helps us make better choices now. We can buy properly processed castor oil. We can be cautious when taking it internally. We can appreciate its thickness for hair or skin, without fearing it because of old myths.

## Legacy in Households

In many families, castor oil has had a place in the medicine cabinet for generations. Grandparents might recall it as a remedy for occasional constipation. Younger folks might have discovered it online as a hair or skin product. Different ages might view it in different ways. But the thread that ties them together is the awareness that castor oil can be a powerful substance if handled right.

For some people, the first time they heard about castor oil was in old movies or stories, where a spoonful was used as a comedic or dreaded moment. This pop culture reference, though, comes from a very real tradition. It may give the impression that castor oil is harsh, but it also serves as a reminder of its potency. That potency has always been part of the story, and it is why people have respected it through the ages.

# CHAPTER 3: CHEMICAL STRUCTURE AND KEY PARTS

Castor oil is often praised for its unusual traits. A key part of why it stands out among plant oils is its main fatty acid, called ricinoleic acid. This chapter will look at what gives castor oil its unique characteristics, from its thick feel to the way it works when applied to the body. We will talk about the main acids found in castor oil, other chemical parts that may be important, and how these parts affect everyday use. By the end of this chapter, you will have a clear explanation of what makes castor oil different and why it has so many uses.

## 1. Overview of Fatty Acids

Most plant oils carry a few common fatty acids, such as oleic acid, linoleic acid, and sometimes linolenic acid. Castor oil shares some of these, but it also has an unusually high level of ricinoleic acid, which is not often found in large amounts in other oils. This difference in fatty acids gives castor oil many of its properties.

- **Oleic Acid:** This is a monounsaturated fatty acid. It is found in olive oil, avocado oil, and many other plant oils. It helps maintain moisture in the skin and can soften hair. Castor oil contains a smaller percentage of oleic acid compared to some other oils.
- **Linoleic Acid:** This is a polyunsaturated fatty acid. It is important for certain skin functions and can help maintain the protective outer layer of the skin. Linoleic acid is also found in safflower oil and sunflower oil. Castor oil has some of this acid, but not as much as certain other oils.
- **Palmitic Acid:** This saturated fatty acid is found in palm oil, animal fats, and many plants. It can provide stability to oils. In castor oil, palmitic acid is present but does not make up a huge fraction.

- **Stearic Acid:** This saturated fatty acid is solid at room temperature and is often used in making soaps and cosmetics. Castor oil holds a small percentage of stearic acid.

---

## 2. Ricinoleic Acid: The Main Star

What makes castor oil special is ricinoleic acid. This fatty acid makes up about 80-90% of the total fatty acid content in castor oil, which is very high compared to other plant oils. Ricinoleic acid has a hydroxyl group in its structure. This means there is an -OH (oxygen-hydrogen) part attached to the fatty acid chain. This feature helps make castor oil thicker and more polar (which influences how it interacts with water or with certain parts of the body).

**Properties of Ricinoleic Acid:**

1. **Thickness and Viscosity:** Ricinoleic acid causes the oil to be more viscous, or thick. This can be useful for applying a protective layer on the skin or hair.
2. **Moisture Retention:** The hydroxyl group helps the oil bond with water molecules, which may allow better moisture retention on the skin.
3. **Possible Soothing Effect:** Some research suggests that ricinoleic acid can reduce minor skin swelling when rubbed on the skin. It may also calm certain types of irritation, which is why some people find castor oil soothing for mild redness or dryness.

Because of this high ricinoleic acid content, castor oil reacts differently in formulas than many other oils. For example, it can mix in ways that create creamier textures in lotions or lip balms. It can also act as a carrier oil that might hold certain added substances well.

---

## 3. Minor Fatty Acids in Castor Oil

While ricinoleic acid is the main feature, there are smaller amounts of other acids that can still be important:

- **Dihydroxystearic Acid:** This acid forms when some of the ricinoleic acid gets converted. It can add thickness and stability to formulas.
- **Others (Trace Amounts):** Castor oil may hold small traces of acids like linolenic acid, eicosenoic acid, and more. Even though they are present in small amounts, they can influence the final feel and behavior of the oil, especially if the oil is refined or partially processed.

Each fatty acid contributes to how the oil smells, feels, and works when used on the skin, hair, or in other applications. While most people may not look at these details, they can be important for those who want to understand exactly why castor oil performs differently than a common cooking oil.

---

## 4. Proteins, Vitamin Content, and Other Components

Castor oil mainly consists of fats, but it can also have tiny amounts of proteins, vitamins, and minerals. Since the oil is extracted from seeds, you might assume it would contain protein. However, most of the protein found in the seeds does not end up in the final product in large amounts. The toxic substance called ricin, which is a protein, is also removed in the refining process. Safe castor oil should not contain any harmful levels of ricin.

- **Vitamins:** Castor oil may contain small amounts of vitamin E, though it is not considered a major source. Vitamin E can help with the shelf life of certain oils, acting as a natural antioxidant.
- **Minerals:** The amounts are usually minimal and do not make castor oil a significant mineral source.
- **Enzymes:** Most enzymes from the seed are not present in the final oil, especially once the oil is filtered.

## 5. Why Thickness Matters

You might wonder why the thickness of castor oil is worth talking about. The thickness affects how it spreads on the skin and how it forms a layer that can lock in moisture. Thinner oils, such as almond oil, run off the skin more easily. Castor oil stays in place longer, which can be useful for certain treatments. For instance, if you want an oil to remain on your feet or scalp overnight, a thick oil might be more suitable.

This thick nature is also why castor oil is often blended with lighter oils in personal care. If you find castor oil too sticky, you can combine it with a lighter oil. The result will likely be easier to spread and wash out. Yet you still get some of the special benefits of ricinoleic acid.

---

## 6. Polarity and Its Effects

One of the lesser-known points about castor oil is that it is more polar than many other fats. Polarity refers to how electrical charges are distributed across a molecule. Because ricinoleic acid has that hydroxyl group, the molecule can interact with water in a limited way. This property is significant when castor oil is used in industrial settings, but it also helps in personal care products. It can act as a partial emulsifier, helping water-based and oil-based ingredients blend a bit better. This is helpful in lotions or creams where water and oil need to stay mixed.

---

## 7. Stability and Shelf Life

Castor oil generally has a good shelf life. This is linked to the fact that ricinoleic acid is more stable than some other unsaturated fatty acids. Oils with high linoleic acid content, such as flaxseed oil, can turn rancid faster if they are not stored properly. Castor oil can last longer without significant change in smell or color, especially if you keep it away from bright light and high heat. Many people store castor oil at room temperature for months or even a couple of years with minimal change.

Still, it is wise to keep an eye (and nose) on the oil. If it develops a strange odor or color, it might be past its best point. Many manufacturers put a "best by" date on the bottle, although castor oil can often stay usable beyond that if it is stored well.

## 8. Interactions with Skin and Hair

**Skin:** When castor oil is applied to the skin, the ricinoleic acid can help form a moist environment that may speed up the skin's natural healing process for minor dryness. The thick layer might protect small cracks or rough spots from further damage. Some people with sensitive skin find it beneficial, but others might experience a breakout if their pores clog easily. Each person's body chemistry is different.

**Hair:** Castor oil can coat the hair shaft, which can reduce the amount of water that escapes. By holding moisture in the hair, castor oil can help the hair feel smooth. There is a common claim that castor oil helps hair grow faster, but there is not a large amount of data to confirm that it directly speeds up hair growth. It might reduce breakage, which can make hair appear fuller over time. The oil also helps reduce friction between strands.

## 9. Soothing Minor Skin Problems

Because of the composition of castor oil, it can calm mild skin complaints. One reason might be that it helps prevent further dryness by keeping an oily layer on the surface. It might also reduce minor itching or redness in some cases. That said, it is still advisable to test a small patch of skin first to see if castor oil is suitable for you. Although it is known to be mild, any oil can cause issues if someone has a personal sensitivity.

## 10. Digestive Action Explained

Many people know castor oil can move the bowels when taken by mouth. The main reason is the ricinoleic acid. When it reaches the small intestine, enzymes break it down into smaller parts. These parts can trigger muscle contractions in the intestines. This can help push waste through. The effect can be quite strong, which is why it is important to use the correct dose. Too much castor oil can lead to cramping or diarrhea. This strong reaction is why castor oil has a reputation as a powerful laxative.

However, in modern times, people often find gentler options for constipation. They might choose fiber supplements or mild over-the-counter products. Castor oil is still an option, but it should be used carefully. One should also note that repeated use of any laxative can cause issues. Over time, the body might become dependent, or you might lose important fluids.

---

## 11. Comparison to Other Oils

To better understand castor oil's chemical structure, we can compare it briefly to a few other popular oils:

- **Olive Oil:** Known for its health benefits, olive oil is rich in oleic acid. It is more fluid than castor oil and does not contain much ricinoleic acid.
- **Coconut Oil:** High in saturated fats, coconut oil is solid in cooler temperatures. While coconut oil is thick when solid, once it melts, it feels lighter than castor oil.
- **Argan Oil:** This oil has a higher amount of vitamin E and is lighter on the skin. It does not have the same laxative effect as castor oil.
- **Jojoba Oil:** Actually a wax ester, jojoba oil is closer to the skin's natural sebum. It is much thinner than castor oil.

These differences underscore castor oil's unique role. If you want a heavier oil that can stay on the surface longer, castor oil is a strong candidate.

## 12. Potential Industrial and Medical Uses

The special structure of ricinoleic acid and the thick texture also make castor oil attractive for certain industrial purposes. It is used to make lubricants for high-performance engines or to produce biodegradable plastics. In some medical settings, castor oil can be a base for protective coatings or certain ointments. Researchers continue to look into new ways to harness the polarity and stability of castor oil. One example is using it as a carrier in drug delivery systems, where medication is mixed into castor oil to help it spread or absorb at a controlled pace.

---

## 13. Factors Influencing the Chemical Makeup

The actual composition of castor oil can vary depending on several factors:

- **Seed Variety:** Different strains of the castor plant may produce oil with slightly varying percentages of ricinoleic acid.
- **Soil and Climate:** The mineral content of the soil and temperature can affect the oil's final makeup.
- **Extraction Method:** Cold-pressed castor oil may hold more of its natural structure, while oils extracted with heat or chemicals can change slightly.
- **Refining Steps:** Additional refining can remove certain components, possibly altering color, scent, or minor fatty acid amounts.

Because of these influences, not every bottle of castor oil will be exactly the same. Still, most high-quality castor oils share the basic profile of being rich in ricinoleic acid and thick in texture.

---

## 14. The Role of pH

Pure fats, including castor oil, do not have a pH in the same sense that water-based solutions do. pH measures hydrogen ions in water. Since castor oil contains little water, discussing pH can be tricky. Some people wonder if castor oil is "acidic" or "alkaline." Technically, we do not measure its pH in the same way we do for water-based substances. Instead, we might talk about its "acid value," which is a different measurement. The acid value refers to the free fatty acid content. Castor oil can have a certain acid value that shows how much of the oil might be broken down into free fatty acids.

In simpler terms, castor oil does not function like a strong acid or base when it is on your skin. It is the structure of the fatty acids, especially ricinoleic acid, that matters more than a standard pH number.

## 15. Emulsifying Properties

An emulsion is a mixture of water and oil. Think of mayonnaise, where oil is blended with an egg and some acid (like vinegar or lemon juice) to create a creamy texture. Castor oil has mild emulsifying properties thanks to its hydroxyl group. While it is not a perfect emulsifier on its own, it can help hold an emulsion together longer than an oil with no hydroxyl groups. This makes it valuable in personal care formulations. When companies make face creams or lotions, castor oil can help keep the product from separating too quickly. It also gives a richer feeling on the skin.

## 16. Soap Making and Saponification

Soap makers often use castor oil in their recipes. In soap making, saponification is the reaction between fats (or oils) and a strong base (often sodium hydroxide) to create soap and glycerin. Castor oil can help boost the lather in a bar of soap and make it feel more conditioning. A bar with too much castor oil might end up sticky, but a moderate amount can produce a pleasant, stable foam.

Ricinoleic acid is key here as well. The hydroxyl group can bond in ways that produce a creamy, stable lather. Some soap enthusiasts find that adding 5-10% castor oil to a soap recipe significantly improves the final bar. Many claim the soap rinses clean yet leaves the skin feeling soft.

## 17. Allergic Reactions and Sensitivities

Although castor oil is often well-tolerated, there is a small chance that some people might be sensitive to it. This could be due to trace impurities, other minor components, or personal skin reactions. Symptoms might include itching, redness, or small bumps. If you suspect you have a reaction, discontinue use and check with a health professional. Overall, true allergies to pure castor oil are not very common, but it is best to test a small area first, especially if you have sensitive skin or a history of allergies.

## 18. Heat Effects on the Structure

When castor oil is heated for refining or for certain cooking purposes (though it is not generally used in common cooking), some changes can occur in its structure. High heat can break some of the fatty acid chains, leading to a change in color or viscosity. That is why cold-pressed castor oil is seen as a good choice for skin and hair. By avoiding high heat, more of the original structure remains intact. However, some processes that use moderate heat may help remove impurities, making the oil clearer or reducing any strong scent. It depends on what purpose you have for the oil.

## 19. Investigations into Ricinoleic Acid's Effects

Scientists have done experiments to see why ricinoleic acid influences the body the way it does. Some studies on lab animals suggest it causes the intestines to contract. Others show it may help soothe skin by reducing certain signals of irritation. Researchers are still exploring the full range of how this fatty acid interacts with cells. While people have used castor oil for a long time, science continues to uncover new details about its chemical behavior. This search may lead to more specialized uses, such as advanced wound dressings or even new medical salves.

## 20. Golden Points About Castor Oil Chemistry

1. **Unique Hydroxyl Group:** Ricinoleic acid has a hydroxyl group, giving castor oil properties not shared by most other plant oils.
2. **High Stability:** It does not go bad as quickly as many oils high in polyunsaturated fats.
3. **Variable Composition:** Factors like seed variety, climate, and processing can change the percentage of minor components.
4. **Industrial Value:** Its polar nature and thickness make it valuable in certain industrial and cosmetic formulations.
5. **Powerful Laxative Action:** Ricinoleic acid triggers bowel movements when used internally in the correct amount.

---

## 21. Practical Lessons from the Chemistry

Understanding the chemistry helps people decide if castor oil is right for their personal use:

- **Skin Soothing:** The thick oil can help shield and soften dry or cracked skin.
- **Hair Coating:** It can coat strands to reduce dryness and friction.
- **Gentle Blending:** Combine it with lighter oils if you find it too sticky.
- **Cautious Internal Use:** If you ever plan to take it by mouth, be mindful of the dose because of its laxative effect.
- **Check Quality:** A properly processed oil should be free from harmful levels of ricin.

This knowledge also guides manufacturers who want to include castor oil in a product. They might design formulas that take advantage of ricinoleic acid's unique structure to get a richer texture or a more stable mixture.

---

## 22. Myths About the Chemical Aspects

There are a few myths floating around regarding castor oil's chemistry:

- **Myth: Castor Oil Contains Ricin:** Ricin is a toxic protein found in raw castor beans, but not in the purified oil if it is correctly processed.
- **Myth: Castor Oil's Thickness Means It Is Full of Waxes:** While castor oil has a thick consistency, it is not a wax like jojoba oil. It is mainly due to the hydroxyl-containing fatty acid.
- **Myth: All Castor Oils Are the Same:** The actual composition can vary, and Jamaican black castor oil is different in color and possibly in minor components due to the roasting process.

## 23. Research Directions

Researchers continue to investigate castor oil for fresh uses. Some labs are looking at how ricinoleic acid might help deliver medication through the skin. Others are exploring if it can reduce certain harmful germs when used in disinfectant products. There is also interest in developing new biodegradable materials from castor oil, given the need to find eco-friendly alternatives to plastics that do not break down well.

## 24. The Bigger Picture

From the standpoint of chemistry, castor oil's main claim to fame is the extraordinary amount of ricinoleic acid. This unusual fatty acid changes how the oil behaves physically and how it can impact the body. While other oils might share certain traits, none has quite the same level of this special acid. This makes castor oil a staple in various tasks, from making soap to treating dry elbows. By knowing about these key parts, users can use castor oil more effectively and confidently.

# CHAPTER 4: HARVESTING AND PROCESSING

To appreciate a final bottle of castor oil, it is helpful to see how the oil is collected and processed. The methods used can change the quality, color, and even the texture of the oil. In this chapter, we will cover how castor plants are grown, what conditions they need, how the seeds are gathered, and how the oil is extracted and refined. We will also explain how safety measures protect users from any harmful parts. By the end of this chapter, you will understand the path from a raw seed in the field to the ready-to-use oil on store shelves.

## 1. Growing Conditions for Castor Plants

The castor plant, *Ricinus communis*, usually grows well in warm regions. It thrives in tropical and subtropical climates, although it can also survive in some temperate zones if the weather is not too cold. This plant prefers well-drained soil, plenty of sunlight, and moderate rainfall.

1. **Soil:** The plant grows best in sandy or loamy soil. Heavy clay soils can cause waterlogging, which can harm the roots.
2. **Temperature:** Ideal temperatures range from about 68°F (20°C) to 86°F (30°C). Prolonged frost can damage or kill the plant.
3. **Water:** While castor plants can handle some dryness, they still need enough water during growth to produce healthy seeds. However, too much water can cause rot.
4. **Sunlight:** Castor plants generally prefer full sun, which helps them produce large leaves and seed pods.

In many countries, farmers grow castor plants on plots of land large or small. The size of these farms can vary widely. Some small-scale farmers grow them for local markets, while large commercial operations produce huge amounts of castor seeds for export.

## 2. Seed Pod Development

One of the distinctive features of the castor plant is its seed pods. These pods are spiky or spiny, resembling small burrs. Inside each pod, there are typically three seeds. The seeds themselves are oval-shaped and can have patterns that range from light brown to speckled. These patterns help give castor seeds an interesting look, but they are also a reminder that they contain dangerous substances if not handled properly.

As the plant matures, the seed pods turn from green to a drier color. Eventually, the pods split open on their own or can be carefully removed by hand or machine. Timing is important, as collecting the seeds too early can lead to low oil yield, while waiting too long may cause the pods to burst and drop seeds on the ground.

## 3. Harvesting Methods

**Manual Harvesting:** In many regions, castor seeds are still picked by hand. Workers wear gloves or other protective gear to avoid contact with the spines on the pods and to avoid any possible irritation. They collect the pods into baskets or sacks, then move them to a processing area. This method allows for careful selection of pods that are fully mature, but it can be labor-intensive and slow.

**Mechanical Harvesting:** Large-scale farms may use machines that shake the plants or strip the seed pods. This can be more efficient, but it may also bring in some unripe pods or extra plant material. Sorting then becomes important. The seeds must be separated from any debris before the oil extraction stage.

In both methods, safety is crucial. Workers must avoid eating or chewing the seeds because they contain ricin, a substance that can be harmful. Once the seeds are collected, they are sent for processing, where the safe oil is extracted and any toxic parts are removed or neutralized.

## 4. Drying and Storing the Seeds

Before oil extraction, the seeds often need to be dried. This can be done by spreading them out in a well-ventilated area, sometimes in the sun, or in dedicated drying facilities. Drying helps lower the moisture content, which can improve oil yield and reduce the risk of mold.

Once dried, the seeds may be stored in sacks or bins until they are ready for pressing. Storage conditions must be dry and cool to prevent spoilage. Some facilities use temperature-controlled storage if they plan to keep seeds for a while. Keeping moisture levels low is a key step, as damp seeds can lead to a lower quality oil or potential fungus issues.

## 5. Traditional Pressing Methods

Historically, people extracted castor oil by hand. They might crush the seeds using a mortar and pestle, then wrap the mash in cloth and press it to squeeze out the oil. In some places, stones or simple wooden presses were used. While this yielded castor oil, the process was slow and might not remove all impurities. The oil could be dark and might carry a strong smell.

Some small communities still use these methods for local needs. The oil produced can be quite thick and might have a "rustic" aroma. It can be used for simple tasks like lamp oil, homemade soap, or folk remedies. However, for larger markets and more refined uses, modern methods are more common now.

## 6. Modern Extraction Techniques

**Cold Pressing:** In cold pressing, seeds are fed into a press machine that squeezes out the oil without using high heat. This method helps preserve the structure of the fatty acids, especially ricinoleic acid. The resulting oil is often labeled "cold-pressed castor oil." It may keep more of its natural color and smell. Some people like cold-pressed oils for skin and hair care because they believe fewer nutrients are lost in the process.

**Expeller Pressing:** This also involves a machine that applies pressure, but it may generate some heat due to friction. The temperature is usually not too high, but it is higher than in cold pressing. Expeller pressing is common and can extract a good amount of oil relatively quickly. The final oil might be slightly darker or have a slightly roasted smell, depending on the exact temperature.

**Solvent Extraction:** In large industrial settings, a chemical solvent (often hexane) can be used to pull oil from the seed mash. Later, the solvent is removed, leaving behind the oil. This method can extract the maximum amount of oil, but it requires more steps to ensure no solvent remains. Some individuals prefer to avoid solvent-extracted oils for personal care, while others do not mind because the final product is usually tested to confirm it is safe.

---

## 7. Filtering and Clarifying

Once the oil is pressed out, it can contain bits of seed or other particles. To get a clearer product, manufacturers filter and clarify the oil. This might involve passing the oil through fine screens or using other filtration materials like diatomaceous earth. The goal is to remove any solids, giving the oil a smoother texture and more stable shelf life.

**Settling Tanks:** Another old-fashioned way is to place the freshly pressed oil in large settling tanks. Over time, heavier particles sink to the bottom, and the clearer oil can be skimmed off the top. This process, while simple, is time-consuming. Modern methods are faster, using pumps and filters to remove particles quickly.

# 8. Refining Steps

Depending on the intended use, castor oil can undergo further refining:

- **Degumming:** This step removes gums and phospholipids. It can help make the oil look clearer and more consistent.
- **Neutralization:** Any free fatty acids can be neutralized with an alkali, reducing acidity. This might be done if the oil has an acid level that is considered too high.
- **Bleaching:** Special clays or activated carbon can be used to lighten the color of the oil. This process is optional, depending on the final product needs.
- **Deodorizing:** Some oils undergo a steam process to remove or reduce strong smells. Castor oil can have a distinct scent, so deodorizing might be used in certain cosmetic or pharmaceutical preparations.

Refining can yield a very neutral product in color and smell. However, some believe that too much refining might reduce certain beneficial compounds. It depends on the balance between the desired purity and preserving as many natural substances as possible.

# 9. Jamaican Black Castor Oil

A special variant, often called Jamaican black castor oil, is made by roasting castor seeds first. The ashes from the roasted hulls are sometimes added back into the oil, giving it a dark color. This oil can have a stronger smell and is quite popular among some groups for hair care. They believe the roasting changes the properties in a beneficial way. Whether this is true or not can be subjective, but it remains a favored style for many who use it on their scalp or hair.

# 10. Safety Measures: Removing Ricin

One of the biggest concerns with castor seeds is the presence of ricin, a potent toxin. Proper processing is designed to ensure ricin does not remain in the final oil. This usually involves:

1. **Heat Treatment:** Applying heat to the seed mash can denature or break down ricin.
2. **Filtering:** Ricin is a protein, so it does not mix well in the pure oil fraction. By carefully removing seed fragments and watery components, most of the ricin is separated from the oil.
3. **Quality Testing:** Reputable producers test their castor oil to confirm it meets safety standards.

As a result, well-made castor oil is considered safe for external and occasional internal uses (within recommended guidelines). Still, swallowing raw seeds is extremely dangerous. This is why castor oil must come from reliable processing facilities that follow all safety rules.

---

# 11. Organic and Fair Trade Options

Some consumers prefer organic castor oil, which means the plants were grown without synthetic pesticides or fertilizers. Organic certification requires proof that the soil and farming practices meet certain standards. Fair trade programs might also exist for castor oil, ensuring that farmers receive a decent income and that working conditions are safe. Choosing organic or fair trade products can be a personal decision, but for those who value eco-friendly and socially responsible products, these labels can be worth looking for.

---

# 12. Storage and Shelf Life After Processing

Once bottled, castor oil can remain stable for quite some time if stored properly. The thick texture and presence of certain natural antioxidants help it resist rancidity. However, light, air, and heat can still break it down gradually. Producers typically advise storing castor oil in a cool, dark place with the cap tightly sealed.

**Common Shelf Life:** Many castor oil products have a listed shelf life of about one to two years. Sometimes, you can use them beyond that if the oil still looks and smells normal. If it becomes cloudy or has an unpleasant odor, it may be time to discard it.

---

## 13. Differences in Color and Aroma

During processing, castor oil can end up with various shades of yellow, light brown, or even dark brown (in the case of Jamaican black castor oil). Some are almost colorless if heavily refined. In addition, the scent can range from mild and nutty to a bit pungent. These differences often reflect the degree of roasting or refining. They do not necessarily mean one is better than the other. It is more about what you prefer or what your intended use demands.

---

## 14. Large-Scale Production and Supply Chain

In regions where castor plants grow well, large factories process huge amounts of seeds. The raw seeds may come from many local farms. They are weighed, tested for moisture and quality, then combined for pressing. The oil is collected in bulk tanks. Some is sold as crude oil for industrial uses (like biodiesel or lubricants). Others are refined further for cosmetics, pharmaceuticals, or food-grade products (though castor oil is not widely used for typical cooking).

The global supply chain can send castor oil across oceans to different continents. It may then be bottled by another company under different brand names. This is why you might see "Product of India" on a bottle sold by a company in the United States. India is currently one of the top producers of castor seeds and castor oil, but other countries also contribute.

## 15. Homemade Extraction: Is It Safe?

Some DIY enthusiasts wonder if they can press their own castor oil from seeds. While it is technically possible, it comes with risks. Handling raw castor seeds requires caution due to ricin. One small mistake could lead to contamination. Also, getting a decent yield without professional equipment can be tough. For these reasons, most people prefer to buy castor oil from a reliable source rather than attempt to make it at home.

## 16. Environmental Impact

Castor plants can be hardy and grow in areas with limited resources. They might not require as much water or fertilizer as some other crops. However, large-scale production could still have environmental consequences, such as land use change or pesticide use if not managed well. On the upside, castor oil is biodegradable and can be used in products that break down more easily than petroleum-based materials. Some see it as a possible source for greener industrial products in the future.

## 17. Quality Control and Testing

Producers usually test the oil for:

- **Acid Value (AV):** Indicates the free fatty acid content.
- **Moisture Content:** Water in the oil can speed up spoilage.
- **Impurities:** Checking for seed particles or dirt.
- **Residual Solvent (if used):** Ensuring the final product has no dangerous solvent levels.
- **Microbial Testing:** Making sure no harmful bacteria or fungus can grow in the oil.

Reputable companies often share such details or will provide them if asked. This helps users know they are getting a clean and safe product.

## 18. Special Processing for Pharmaceutical-Grade Oil

Pharmaceutical-grade castor oil undergoes stricter checks. It must meet specific standards for purity set by official pharmacopeias. These guidelines cover everything from the maximum allowed acid value to the absence of contaminants. This level of quality is required if the oil will be used in medicines or medical treatments. Some eye drops or certain injections might use castor oil as a carrier, so it has to be extremely pure.

## 19. Observing Changes in Different Batches

Even if you buy the same brand, there can be slight changes between batches. The color could be slightly more yellow or a bit clearer. The viscosity might vary if the seeds came from a different region. Usually, these differences do not affect the oil's overall function. Yet, if you notice a dramatic change, you might want to contact the company or check if the oil is still good.

## 20. From Seed to Your Shelf: A Brief Recap

1. **Castor Plants Grown:** Farmers plant castor seeds in suitable climates. The plants mature, producing spiny seed pods.
2. **Harvesting:** Pods are gathered by hand or machine. Workers must be careful, since the seeds contain toxic substances.
3. **Drying and Sorting:** The seeds are dried to reduce moisture and sorted to remove dirt or bad seeds.
4. **Pressing or Extraction:** The seeds are pressed or treated with solvent to release their oil. Cold-pressing, expeller pressing, or solvent extraction may be used.
5. **Filtering and Refining:** The oil is filtered to remove solids, and it may be degummed, bleached, or deodorized if needed.

6. **Bottling:** The final product is packaged in bottles or containers. Some might be labeled "cold-pressed," "organic," or "Jamaican black."
7. **Quality Check:** The manufacturer tests the oil to ensure it is safe and meets desired standards.
8. **Distribution:** Bottles are shipped to stores or sold online. They end up in households for use in skin care, hair care, home remedies, and more.

---

## 21. Practical Tips for Selecting the Right Castor Oil

- **Check Labels:** Look for terms like "cold-pressed" or "expeller-pressed" if you want less processed oil.
- **Decide on Color and Smell:** A lighter oil may indicate more refining, which some prefer. Jamaican black castor oil is darker and stronger in smell.
- **Review Brand Reputation:** Buy from companies that explain how they process and test their oil.
- **Look for Certificates (if desired):** If organic or fair trade is important to you, see if the product displays those certifications.
- **Consider Your Use:** If you plan to use castor oil in homemade skin products, you might prefer a certain texture or aroma.

---

## 22. Storage at Home

Once you have a bottle of castor oil, keep it in a cool, dark spot. A bathroom cabinet might be fine if it does not get too hot or humid. You can also keep it in the refrigerator, but remember it will become thicker in cold temperatures. Always keep the lid tightly closed to block air from getting in. If you have a large container, you may want to pour a smaller amount into a smaller bottle for regular use. This helps keep the main supply fresher for a longer time.

## 23. Safety for Household Use

- **Label Clearly:** If you keep castor oil in a different bottle, label it to avoid confusion.
- **Keep Away from Children:** While normal external use is generally safe, swallowing large amounts can cause strong laxative effects. Children should not handle castor oil unsupervised.
- **Watch for Reactions:** If you notice any rash or itching after using castor oil on your skin, stop using it and consider speaking with a professional.
- **Measure Carefully if Swallowed:** If you plan to take a small amount of castor oil for digestive reasons, follow the correct dosage. Too much can be risky.

---

## 24. Ongoing Studies on Farming Methods

Agricultural experts continue to explore how to grow castor plants in ways that use fewer chemicals and preserve the soil. Some are testing intercropping methods, where castor plants are grown alongside other crops. This might reduce pests naturally and improve biodiversity. Others are trying to develop new castor plant varieties that produce higher oil yields or are more resistant to disease. Such research may lower production costs and make the oil more accessible worldwide.

# CHAPTER 5: HEALTHY SKIN SUPPORT

Castor oil has a long record of being a simple yet helpful option for skin care. While some people use modern creams and lotions, others turn to castor oil for its thickness and the special parts it holds. In this chapter, we will explore how castor oil can support different parts of the skin, from dryness on heels to the delicate surface on the face. We will look at how to apply it, how often to use it, and some lesser-known ways to get the most out of its benefits. By the end, you should have a wide range of tips to help you add castor oil to your skin care routine in a safe way.

## 1. Why Skin Health Matters

Skin is the body's biggest organ. It acts as a shield against outside dangers like germs and harsh weather. It also helps the body hold moisture and get rid of waste through sweat. Healthy skin often looks fresh and can play a part in a person's sense of confidence. Taking care of skin involves more than just washing it; it involves giving it the moisture and nourishment it needs, avoiding too much sun or harsh chemicals, and picking the right products for your skin type.

## 2. Key Reasons Castor Oil Can Help the Skin

Castor oil can help keep skin healthy for many reasons:

1. **Thickness:** Because it is thick, castor oil does not run off the skin too quickly. This can help form a temporary barrier that keeps moisture from escaping.

2. **Unique Fatty Acid Content:** Ricinoleic acid may soothe mild redness or dryness. It can also help the skin hold on to its natural moisture.
3. **Protective Layer:** A small amount of castor oil on the skin's surface can reduce friction, which might help avoid minor skin cracks or small sores.
4. **Ease of Mixing:** If castor oil feels too heavy, you can blend it with lighter oils like grape seed oil or sweet almond oil. This can make it easier to spread over bigger areas of the body.

## 3. Types of Skin Issues Castor Oil May Help

1. **Dry or Flaky Areas:** Castor oil's thick texture can help soften parts of the skin that tend to become flaky, such as elbows and knees.
2. **Rough Hands and Cuticles:** People who do a lot of work with their hands may find relief by rubbing in a small amount of castor oil.
3. **Chapped Lips:** A tiny dab of castor oil can help protect lips from dryness, though you should be careful not to lick it off.
4. **Minor Skin Blemishes:** Some individuals claim castor oil helps fade the look of small spots over time. This is not guaranteed for everyone, but it may work for some.
5. **Light Wrinkles:** Because castor oil keeps moisture in, it can help the skin appear plumper, which may reduce the look of fine lines.

It is important to note that serious skin conditions should be handled by a health professional. Castor oil might help with mild concerns, but it should not replace medical advice or prescribed products.

## 4. Simple Skin Care Routine with Castor Oil

A basic way to use castor oil for skin is to follow a short routine once or twice a day:

1. **Cleanse:** Wash your face or the area with a mild, non-drying soap or cleanser. Rinse with lukewarm water and gently pat it dry with a soft towel.
2. **Apply a Small Amount:** Place a drop or two of castor oil in your palm. Rub your hands together to warm it slightly. This makes it easier to spread.
3. **Massage Lightly:** Gently rub the oil onto the skin in small circles. Focus on areas that need extra moisture or feel rough.
4. **Wait:** Allow the oil to sit on the skin for a few minutes so it can soak in. If the skin looks or feels oily after a while, use a clean towel to dab away extra oil.
5. **Optional Step - Mix with Another Product:** You can combine castor oil with your usual moisturizer to enhance the moisturizing effect. Blend them in your hands before applying.

---

## 5. Tips for Facial Use

When using castor oil on the face, caution is key. Some people's pores might clog easily, especially in the T-zone (forehead, nose, and chin). Here are some ideas:

- **Patch Test First:** Apply a small amount of castor oil on your jawline or near your ear. Wait a day or two and see if you get any bumps. If not, it is probably safe for regular use.
- **Avoid Overuse:** Too much castor oil on the face can leave a sticky layer that may trap dirt. Use only a small drop, and see how your skin reacts over time.
- **Combine with Lighter Oils:** If pure castor oil is too thick for your face, consider mixing it 1:1 with jojoba oil or argan oil. This can balance out the heaviness.
- **Night-Time Application:** Many people prefer to use castor oil on their face at night. That way, it has time to sit on the skin, and any extra can be wiped off in the morning.
- **Remove Makeup First:** Always remove makeup and wash your face before applying castor oil to allow better absorption.

## 6. Addressing Dry Patches and Cracked Skin

Dry patches can appear on the feet, especially around the heels, as well as on hands and elbows. Castor oil may help ease these areas:

1. **Soak First:** If treating feet, try soaking them in warm water for about 10 minutes. You can add a bit of Epsom salt if you like.
2. **Dry Thoroughly:** Pat your feet dry with a towel.
3. **Rub in Oil:** Take a small amount of castor oil and rub it into the rough or cracked areas.
4. **Cover with Socks:** Put on a pair of clean cotton socks to keep the oil from rubbing off on the floor or sheets. This also locks in the moisture.
5. **Repeat as Needed:** Doing this once or twice a week can soften tough patches over time.

This approach can also be used on elbows, knees, or knuckles. Some people use a small bandage to cover the area if it is a small crack. If the dryness is severe or painful, see a health professional.

---

## 7. Dealing with Minor Skin Blemishes

Though results vary, some individuals say that castor oil helps reduce the look of small blemishes or discolored areas:

- **Targeted Application:** Use a cotton swab to dab a tiny bit of castor oil on the blemish. Massage gently and let it sit.
- **Overnight Treatment:** If possible, apply at night and cover the area with a small bandage or cloth to keep the oil in place.
- **Patience:** Changes might not appear overnight. It can take days or weeks of regular use to see any difference.

If you have serious skin discoloration or scars, it might be best to consult a health professional for more advanced treatments.

## 8. Castor Oil Packs for the Abdomen or Joints

Castor oil packs are more often talked about for deeper support (for example, placing them on the abdomen to possibly support digestion), but they can also support the skin in those areas. Here is a quick overview:

1. **Choose a Soft Cloth:** Cotton flannel is often used.
2. **Warm the Oil:** Gently heat the castor oil by placing the bottle in a bowl of warm water. Do not boil it or place it directly on high heat.
3. **Soak the Cloth:** Pour enough oil on the cloth so that it is saturated but not dripping.
4. **Apply to Skin:** Lay the cloth on the area you want to cover.
5. **Cover:** Some people cover the cloth with plastic wrap or a towel to prevent mess.
6. **Heat:** If desired, place a heating pad or hot water bottle on top, watching the temperature to avoid burns.
7. **Rest:** Leave the pack on for 30 to 60 minutes. Then remove and wipe away any extra oil.

Although this method is sometimes used for deeper reasons than just skin health, the skin in that area can still benefit from the extended contact with the oil.

---

## 9. Mixing Castor Oil with Other Ingredients

Castor oil can be combined with different items to create homemade skin treatments. Some popular mixes:

1. **Sugar or Salt Scrub:** Mix equal parts castor oil and sugar (or salt) in a small bowl. Use this to gently scrub rough areas, then rinse and pat dry. This can help remove dead skin cells, letting the oil sink in better.
2. **Honey and Castor Oil Mask:** Blend a teaspoon of honey with a teaspoon of castor oil. Apply to the face or rough spots for 10-15 minutes. The stickiness of honey can trap moisture, and castor oil adds extra smoothness.

3. **Aloe Vera Gel Mixture:** Combine one part castor oil with two parts aloe vera gel. Aloe vera can cool the skin, and castor oil can lock in moisture. This might help people with mild irritation, although results vary.
4. **Essential Oils:** A few drops of a mild essential oil (like lavender or chamomile) can be added to castor oil to improve the smell. However, be sure to do a patch test, as essential oils can sometimes irritate sensitive skin.

---

## 10. Preventing and Soothing Minor Sunburn

While castor oil is not a sunscreen and will not block harmful rays, it might help soothe mild sunburn:

- **Cool Water Rinse:** First, cool down the burned area with room-temperature water.
- **Pat Dry:** Use a soft towel to dry, avoiding harsh rubbing that can worsen the skin.
- **Apply Thin Layer:** Rub a light layer of castor oil on the sunburned area to help keep moisture in.
- **Monitor Skin Reaction:** If the burn is serious or if the skin blisters, seek medical help rather than relying on home remedies.

---

## 11. Using Castor Oil for Facial Massage

Facial massages can help muscles relax and temporarily improve blood flow. Some like to use castor oil for this purpose due to its thickness:

1. **Clean Face:** Start with a clean face so that dirt does not get massaged deeper into the pores.
2. **Warm the Oil:** Put a few drops on your fingertips and rub them together.
3. **Gentle Movements:** Use slow, gentle upward circles, starting at the chin and moving outward. Take care around the eyes, as the skin is delicate.

4. **Wipe or Rinse:** After a few minutes, blot away extra oil with a soft cloth. You can also wash your face gently if you prefer not to have oil sit on your skin.

This can be a short self-care practice at the end of the day. Some also add a mild essential oil, but only if they are not sensitive to scents.

---

## 12. Potential Downsides and Warnings

- **Risk of Clogged Pores:** Castor oil can clog pores for some individuals, especially if used in large amounts on the face. Testing first can help you see if your skin reacts badly.
- **Possible Allergic Reactions:** Though rare, some people might have a reaction to castor oil. If you see redness, itching, or bumps, stop use and rinse the area.
- **Staining of Clothes:** Because castor oil is thick, it can leave noticeable stains. Wear older clothes or cover your skin with a towel if you are applying it in places that touch fabric.
- **Overuse on Open Wounds:** While castor oil can help skin around minor cuts, be cautious about placing it directly on open, serious wounds without professional advice.

---

## 13. Supporting Nails and Cuticles

Healthy nails also depend on good skin care around the nail bed. Castor oil can be helpful for:

1. **Cuticle Softening:** After a shower, rub a tiny drop of castor oil on each cuticle. Let it soak in for a minute. This can make it easier to push back the cuticles if that is part of your routine.
2. **Dry or Peeling Nails:** If your nails peel or crack easily, try massaging a drop of castor oil into each nail in the evening. This might help lock in moisture.

3. **Nail Growth:** While research does not confirm that castor oil directly speeds up nail growth, many people feel it protects the nail surface, helping reduce breakage.

This can be especially useful for those who frequently wash their hands or use cleaning products that dry out the nails and skin.

---

## 14. Facial Steam with Castor Oil

Some people enjoy a facial steam to open pores and let treatments sink in:

1. **Heat Water:** Bring a pot of water to a gentle boil, then remove from heat.
2. **Add a Few Drops of Castor Oil:** You can place a few drops into the water. Alternatively, you can apply a very thin layer of castor oil to your face beforehand.
3. **Steam with Caution:** Hold your face about 8-12 inches away from the steaming water. You can drape a towel over your head to trap steam, but be sure not to get too close to avoid burns.
4. **Time Frame:** Steam for about 5 minutes.
5. **Pat Dry:** Gently pat your face dry. Then, if you like, apply more castor oil or your favorite moisturizer.

Steaming can help remove some surface dirt, but do not overdo it, especially if you have sensitive skin. Once or twice a week is usually enough.

---

## 15. Homemade Balms and Ointments

Castor oil is common in homemade balms because it can give a nice thickness. Here is a simple balm idea:

- **Ingredients:** 2 tablespoons of castor oil, 2 tablespoons of beeswax pastilles, 1 tablespoon of another light oil like coconut or olive.
- **Process:**

1. Melt the beeswax in a double boiler on low heat.
2. Stir in the castor oil and the extra oil until it is all combined.
3. Remove from heat and carefully pour into small containers.
4. Let it cool.

Once the balm sets, you can use it on rough spots, lips, or cuticles. The beeswax helps thicken the mixture, while castor oil provides strong moisture retention. Label the container and store it in a cool place. This is just one basic recipe; you can adjust the ratio to get a consistency you like.

---

## 16. Supporting General Skin Comfort

Many individuals who have itchy or tight skin from dryness might find comfort in castor oil rubs:

- **Whole Body Application:** After a bath or shower, lightly towel off and apply a thin layer of castor oil to arms, legs, and torso. Then, gently pat away extra oil with a towel.
- **Mixed with Lotion:** If pure castor oil is too sticky, mix it in your hands with your usual body lotion. This might make it easier to apply.
- **Calming Mild Itch:** Because castor oil locks in moisture, it may help calm mild itchiness tied to dryness.

If the itching or dryness is severe or is from a medical condition, it is best to get professional advice. Castor oil can help as a simple support measure, but might not solve the underlying cause.

---

## 17. How to Store Castor Oil Used for Skin Care

If you only plan to use castor oil on your skin, you do not need a food-grade product. You still want a pure product that is free from pollutants, though. Look for a well-known brand, and keep the bottle sealed in a cool, dim spot. Some people pour small amounts into a travel-size bottle, so they do not expose the full container to air every time they open it. This can keep the main supply fresh.

## 18. Extra Steps for Better Skin

While castor oil can help the skin in many ways, remember that a complete approach to skin health also includes:

- **Proper Hydration:** Drinking enough water helps support skin health from the inside.
- **Balanced Diet:** Eating foods with vitamins and minerals (like vitamin C, vitamin E, and healthy fats) can help the skin stay strong.
- **Sun Protection:** Using sunscreen or protective clothing is important. Castor oil does not replace sunscreen.
- **Regular Cleaning Routines:** Washing off sweat, dirt, and makeup gently can keep pores from getting blocked.

Castor oil is an external product, so pairing it with healthy daily habits can make a bigger difference.

## 19. A Look at Some Myths

- **"Castor Oil Cures All Skin Problems Instantly":** This is not accurate. Castor oil can help lock in moisture and may assist with minor issues, but it is not a miracle cure for major skin conditions.
- **"Putting More Oil Will Help Faster":** Overusing castor oil might lead to greasy skin or clogged pores, especially on the face. Start small.
- **"Allergic Reactions Never Happen":** While rare, they can happen. A patch test is still a good idea.

## 20. Combining Castor Oil with Other Oils for Different Skin Types

- **Oily Skin:** Blend 1 part castor oil with 2 parts a lighter oil like grape seed or jojoba. This can reduce the heaviness.
- **Dry Skin:** Blend equal parts castor oil and almond oil. This helps spread the castor oil more easily over large, dry areas.
- **Sensitive Skin:** Test a small amount of castor oil mixed with a soothing carrier like coconut oil. Watch for any redness.

Everyone's skin is unique, so a mix that works for one person might not be as good for another. Experiment with small amounts until you find a balance that feels comfortable.

---

## 21. Common Mistakes to Avoid

1. **Using Dirty Hands:** Always wash your hands before applying castor oil to keep germs out.
2. **Applying on Unclean Skin:** If there is dirt or makeup on your skin, the oil might trap it, which can lead to breakouts.
3. **Too Much Pressure When Rubbing:** Rubbing too hard can cause irritation. A gentle touch is best.
4. **Ignoring Expiry Dates:** While castor oil can last a while, always check for changes in smell or color if it has been stored for a long time.
5. **Not Following Up on Serious Concerns:** If you have a recurring rash, large skin cracks, or other concerns that do not improve, see a professional.

---

## 22. Seasonal Considerations

- **Winter:** This season can be very drying to the skin, especially in places where indoor heating reduces humidity. Applying castor oil to damp skin after a bath might help keep moisture locked in.
- **Summer:** If you sweat a lot, a heavy oil might feel too sticky. Consider using less castor oil or mixing it with a bigger amount of a lighter oil.

- **Transitions (Spring and Fall):** Changes in temperature and humidity can affect the skin. Adjust how much castor oil you use based on how your skin feels during these changes.

---

## 23. Caring for Sensitive Areas

- **Under the Eyes:** The skin under the eyes is thin. Use a tiny drop of castor oil, and gently dab it with your ring finger. Avoid getting oil in the eyes. If you do, rinse gently with water.
- **Around the Mouth:** If you have laugh lines or dryness at the corners of your mouth, you can dab a small bit of castor oil there. Be sure not to ingest it.
- **Neck:** The neck can show signs of aging or dryness. If you apply castor oil there, remember to massage upward, and do not overapply since clothes can rub it off.

---

## 24. Homemade Skin Softening Treatment

Here is a simple method you can try at home for hands or feet:

- **Items Needed:** A clean bowl, warm water, mild soap, a towel, castor oil, and cotton gloves or socks.
- **Steps:**
    1. Wash your hands or feet with mild soap and warm water.
    2. Pat them mostly dry, but leave them slightly damp.
    3. Apply a few drops of castor oil and rub thoroughly over the skin.
    4. Put on the cotton gloves or socks.
    5. Relax for 15-30 minutes. Some people like to do this at night and sleep with them on.
    6. Remove the gloves or socks and see if the skin feels softer.

Doing this a few times a week can help maintain smoothness in problem areas.

# CHAPTER 6: HAIR AND SCALP CARE

Castor oil is widely used for hair and scalp care. Its thickness, moisture-locking ability, and rich fatty acid content can help keep hair strands smooth. Many people say their hair feels stronger and looks shinier after using castor oil. But is it right for everyone, and how exactly should it be applied? This chapter will explain different methods, possible benefits, and any risks linked to using castor oil for hair and scalp care. Whether you have curly, straight, thick, or fine hair, there may be a way to use castor oil that fits your needs.

## 1. Why Consider Castor Oil for Hair?

Hair can get damaged by heat tools, hair dyes, rough brushing, or simply the stress of daily life. The scalp itself can become dry, itchy, or produce too much oil. Castor oil's traits may address some of these points:

- **Thickness:** Castor oil can coat the hair shaft, possibly keeping moisture in and protecting strands from damage.
- **Possible Reduced Breakage:** When hair strands are lubricated with oil, they may rub against each other less, leading to fewer splits.
- **Scalp Moisture:** A small amount of castor oil can help a dry scalp feel better, though too much oil might cause a heavy feeling.
- **Easy to Blend:** If castor oil is too thick, you can mix it with a lighter oil (like coconut or olive) to get a product that spreads more easily.

## 2. Different Ways to Use Castor Oil on Hair

1. **Pre-Shampoo Treatment:** Some apply castor oil to dry hair and scalp before washing. They let it sit for 15-30 minutes, then shampoo. This can help lessen the drying effects of shampoo.

2. **Deep Conditioning Mask:** Others combine castor oil with a hair mask or conditioner, leaving it on for a longer period (up to an hour). They might wrap their hair in a warm towel to help the oil penetrate better.
3. **Scalp Massage:** Applying a small amount of castor oil to the fingertips and gently massaging the scalp can help loosen flakes and improve overall comfort.
4. **Leave-In Treatment:** A tiny drop of castor oil can be used as a leave-in product on the ends of hair to reduce frizz. However, you must use very little to avoid greasy-looking hair.

## 3. Handling Different Hair Types

- **Curly or Coily Hair:** These types often benefit from extra moisture. Castor oil can help reduce frizz and keep curls looking more defined. People with these hair types sometimes apply castor oil at night, braid or twist the hair, and wash or style in the morning.
- **Straight and Fine Hair:** Castor oil might feel heavy if used in large amounts. A small drop rubbed between palms and then applied mostly to the ends may be enough. Mixing the oil with a lighter product might help avoid a weighted look.
- **Wavy Hair:** A balanced approach is best. Wavy hair can sometimes be dry at the ends and oily near the scalp. Focusing castor oil on the mid-lengths and ends might be a good choice.
- **Color-Treated Hair:** Some say castor oil helps keep dyed hair from drying out, but it may not prevent color from fading. Test a small section first if you are worried about any reaction with hair dye.

## 4. Step-by-Step Hair Mask with Castor Oil

Here is a simple hair mask you can do at home:

1. **Gather Supplies:** Castor oil, a lighter oil (optional), a bowl, a spoon, a shower cap or plastic wrap, and a towel.

2. **Mix the Oil:** If castor oil is too thick for you, blend 2 tablespoons of castor oil with 1 tablespoon of coconut or olive oil in a bowl. Adjust as needed for your hair length.
3. **Section Your Hair:** Part your hair into manageable sections. This helps with even distribution.
4. **Apply to Scalp and Hair:** Dip your fingertips into the oil mixture and gently massage it onto the scalp. Move down the hair shafts all the way to the ends.
5. **Cover:** Put on a shower cap or wrap plastic around your head to hold in heat and keep from making a mess.
6. **Wait:** Relax for 20-60 minutes, depending on how deep you want the treatment to be. Some people apply a warm towel over the cap for extra effect.
7. **Rinse and Wash:** Use a gentle shampoo to rinse out the oil. You may need to shampoo twice if the oil is still noticeable.
8. **Condition (Optional):** If your hair feels dry, follow with a light conditioner. Otherwise, you can skip it because the castor oil may have already provided moisture.
9. **Style:** Let your hair air-dry or style as usual.

Repeat this treatment once a week or every other week, depending on your hair's needs.

---

## 5. Tips for Scalp Massage

A scalp massage can feel good and may help reduce stress:

- **Small Amounts:** Start with a dime-sized amount of castor oil. Add more only if you need it.
- **Gentle Pressure:** Use your fingertips (not your nails) to move in circular motions.
- **Focus on Key Areas:** Pay special attention to areas that feel dry or itchy.
- **Short Sessions:** A 3-5 minute massage is enough for most people.
- **Wash If Needed:** If your scalp feels too oily afterward, rinse with a mild shampoo. If you like a bit of oil on the scalp, you can leave it in.

## 6. Possible Help with Scalp Issues

Some claim that castor oil can help with dandruff or mild scalp flaking. While it is not a proven cure for these conditions, it might reduce dryness. If dandruff is caused by a fungus, certain studies suggest that ricinoleic acid in castor oil may limit some fungal growth in lab tests. However, serious scalp issues often need specialized products or a visit to a dermatologist. Castor oil can be one part of a personal scalp routine, but watch for any signs of increased itching or redness.

## 7. Addressing Hair Loss Worries

There are many claims online that castor oil can stop hair loss or make hair grow faster. Solid research on these claims is limited. However, there is a chance that the oil can reduce breakage and keep hair looking fuller. By keeping hair moisturized and reducing split ends, hair might reach a longer length over time because it is not breaking as much. Still, if you have severe hair loss, talk to a professional, as it might be linked to hormones, genetics, or medical conditions.

## 8. Caring for Braids or Protective Styles

People who wear braids, twists, or other long-term protective styles might use castor oil to keep the scalp moisturized. When hair is braided close to the scalp, dryness or flaking might happen if the scalp is not cared for:

- **Focus on Scalp:** Use a nozzle bottle or a small dropper to place a small amount of castor oil along the scalp in between braided sections.
- **Massage Gently:** Do not disturb the braids too much. Light taps or small circular motions with a fingertip can help the oil spread.

- **Avoid Product Buildup:** Try not to overuse products, or the scalp and braids can become sticky. A weekly or bi-weekly light application might be enough.

---

## 9. Combining Castor Oil with Other Hair-Friendly Ingredients

1. **Aloe Vera Gel:** Some blend aloe vera gel with castor oil for a scalp-soothing mask. Aloe vera adds a cooling effect, while the castor oil can lock in moisture.
2. **Honey:** Known for its humectant properties, honey can attract moisture. Mixing it with castor oil might help very dry hair.
3. **Egg Yolk:** Some homemade hair masks include raw egg yolk for protein. If you try this, rinse with cool water to avoid cooking the egg in your hair.
4. **Essential Oils:** Adding a drop or two of oils like rosemary or lavender may freshen the smell. But be cautious with essential oils if you have allergies or a sensitive scalp.

---

## 10. Overnight Treatments

Leaving castor oil on overnight can give a deeper result for those with extremely dry or curly hair:

- **Protect Pillows:** Wear a shower cap or wrap your hair in a satin scarf to prevent oil from staining your bedding.
- **Less Is More:** Only use a moderate amount of oil so it does not drip.
- **Wash in the Morning:** Shampoo and condition as normal. The hair may feel softer, but if it seems greasy, a second wash might be needed.

Be sure overnight oiling feels comfortable. If it bothers your sleep, you can choose a shorter treatment time.

---

## 11. Preventing Split Ends

Split ends happen when the hair shaft becomes weak or frayed. While castor oil cannot fix splits that already exist, it can help keep the ends of the hair lubricated. This might slow down more splitting:

- **Trim Regularly:** Even if you use oils, getting rid of damaged ends is important.
- **Apply to Ends:** Focus on the last 2-3 inches of your hair with a small amount of castor oil. This can help limit dryness and breakage.
- **Avoid Heat Tools:** Excessive blow-drying or flat ironing can undo the benefits of oil treatments. If you must use heat, apply a heat protectant product.

---

## 12. Using Castor Oil for Shine

If you want to add shine to your hair without making it look oily:

1. **Tiny Amount:** After styling, warm a drop of castor oil between your palms.
2. **Smooth Over Top Layer:** Gently glide your hands over the surface of your hair, focusing on flyaways. Avoid the roots unless your scalp is very dry.
3. **Check in Natural Light:** Step into natural light to see if you need more. Too much can make hair look heavy or greasy.

---

## 13. Possible Drawbacks for Hair and Scalp

- **Over-Oiling:** Applying too much castor oil can lead to flat, greasy-looking hair that is hard to wash out.
- **Scalp Buildup:** If you apply castor oil often but do not clean the scalp thoroughly, you might get buildup. This can clog follicles and lead to itchiness.
- **Allergies:** Though uncommon, some people could have a reaction. If your scalp becomes red or irritated, stop use.

- **Time-Consuming Cleansing:** Because it is thick, you may need multiple washes to remove all the oil, which can be time-consuming.

---

## 14. Tips for Easier Washing

If you find castor oil difficult to remove from your hair, try these tricks:

- **Pre-Shampoo Mix:** Blend the castor oil with a lighter oil. This can make it easier to rinse.
- **Use Warm Water:** Warm water (not too hot) can help loosen the oil.
- **Apply Shampoo on Dry Hair First:** Before wetting your hair, rub shampoo into the oiled areas. This can help break down the oil. Then add water and lather as usual.
- **Use a Clarifying Shampoo Once in a While:** If you are a regular user of heavy oils, a clarifying shampoo once every few weeks can help remove buildup.

---

## 15. Hair Growth Myths vs. Reality

Some marketing claims suggest castor oil can make hair grow one inch per month or more, which is not proven. Average hair growth is around half an inch per month. Castor oil may help reduce breakage, making hair look healthier, which might give the impression of faster growth. But it does not change your genetics or the growth cycle of the hair follicle. If your hair is not growing due to a medical condition, it is best to talk with a professional.

---

## 16. Special Uses: Eyebrows and Eyelashes

Many people also use castor oil on eyebrows or eyelashes to help them appear thicker:

- **Eyebrows:** Dip a clean spoolie or cotton swab in a small amount of castor oil, then brush it along the eyebrows. Wipe away excess to avoid dripping.
- **Eyelashes:** Using a clean mascara wand, lightly coat the lashes with castor oil. Be very careful not to get oil in your eyes.
- **Frequency:** Once a day (often at night) is enough. You do not want to risk irritation from too much oil near the eyes.
- **Results:** Some see a slight improvement in the look of their brows and lashes, but individual results vary. This will not cause overnight growth.

---

## 17. Using Castor Oil for Beards or Facial Hair

Some men and women apply castor oil to facial hair to keep it looking tidy and less prone to dryness:

- **Clean Beard First:** Wash your beard or facial hair with a mild cleanser.
- **Dry Thoroughly:** Pat it dry with a towel.
- **Apply Oil:** Take a small drop of castor oil in your palms, rub them together, then smooth over the beard or mustache.
- **Comb or Brush:** Use a beard comb or brush to distribute the oil evenly.
- **Avoid Overdoing It:** Too much oil can make the hair look greasy or cause irritation on the skin beneath.

---

## 18. Simple DIY Hair Serum

If you want a homemade hair serum with castor oil:

- **Ingredients:** 1 tablespoon castor oil, 1 tablespoon argan oil, 2 tablespoons aloe vera gel (pure), and a small pump bottle.
- **Method:**
    1. Mix all ingredients in a small bowl.
    2. Transfer to the pump bottle.

3. Shake before each use.
- **Use:** After washing and towel-drying hair, apply a small pump of serum to your palms and distribute through the ends of your hair. This might add shine without overwhelming the roots. Store this mixture in a cool, dry place for up to a month.

---

## 19. Protecting Children's Hair

If you plan to use castor oil on a child's hair:

- **Check for Sensitivity:** Children's scalps can be delicate. Use a smaller amount and watch for any reaction.
- **Avoid Eyes and Mouth:** Children can move suddenly, so be careful not to get oil in their eyes.
- **Gentle Washing:** Use a mild, child-friendly shampoo to remove the oil.
- **Frequency:** Once a week or every two weeks might be enough, depending on dryness.

---

## 20. Maintaining a Routine

A consistent hair care plan is more effective than random treatments. If you want to see long-term changes in the look or feel of your hair, make a simple schedule:

- **Weekly Deep Condition:** Use a castor oil-based mask once a week.
- **Daily or Every Other Day Moisture:** If your hair is dry, apply a small drop of castor oil to ends or comb it through after showering.
- **Trim as Needed:** Keep those split ends in check by getting regular trims.
- **Monitor Results:** If your hair seems weighed down or your scalp feels greasy, reduce how often you use the oil or switch up the ratio of oils in your mixture.

## 21. Watching Out for Product Claims

Not all hair products labeled "castor oil" are pure. Some might have added fragrances or fillers. If you want a pure product, read labels and look for words like "100% castor oil" or "pure castor oil." If you see a long list of other ingredients, it may be a blend. That is not always bad, but it depends on whether you want just castor oil or a mix.

---

## 22. Seasonal Concerns for Hair

- **Cold Winters:** The air can be dry, and indoor heating can remove moisture. A weekly castor oil mask could help keep hair from becoming brittle.
- **Humid Summers:** High humidity might make hair frizzy. Use very little castor oil to avoid adding extra weight.
- **Sweaty Seasons:** If you sweat often or swim in pools, you may need to shampoo more often, which can strip hair. A light castor oil pre-shampoo treatment might help offset dryness.

---

## 23. Hair Styling with Castor Oil

If you style your hair with heat or tight braids, consider these points:

- **Before Heat Styling:** Use a dedicated heat protectant, not just castor oil. Oil alone does not protect fully against high heat.
- **Braid Outs or Twist Outs:** Castor oil can be applied before braiding or twisting to help define the pattern.
- **Low Manipulation:** Oiled hair might be easier to detangle, reducing breakage during styling. Use a wide-tooth comb or your fingers.

---

## 24. Choosing Quality Oil for Hair

Factors that may matter:

- **Cold-Pressed:** Some believe cold-pressed oil retains more nutrients.
- **Refined vs. Unrefined:** Refined oil might have fewer impurities, but unrefined could have a stronger smell.
- **Jamaican Black Castor Oil:** This variant can be heavier, with a roasted smell. Some claim it gives better results for thick hair, though personal preferences vary.
- **Brand Reputation:** Look for reviews or company information about sourcing and processing.

## 25. Final Words on Hair and Scalp Care

Castor oil can be a simple and flexible way to care for hair. Its thickness can help protect strands, add shine, and soothe the scalp. But it is not a magical fix for major hair problems. If you are dealing with severe hair loss or scalp concerns, it is best to seek help from a qualified person. Otherwise, castor oil can fit well into a moderate, consistent hair care routine.

In the next chapter, we will look at castor oil's role in digestive support. Castor oil has a well-known effect on the bowels when taken by mouth, though it must be used carefully. We will go over traditional uses, modern thoughts, and safety rules so you can make an informed choice about whether this approach is suitable for you.

# CHAPTER 7: DIGESTIVE SUPPORT

Castor oil is known for its strong effect on the bowels when taken by mouth. For many years, people in different places have used it in small amounts to help with occasional constipation. Some families have passed down tips about swallowing a spoonful of castor oil to "get things moving." But while this method can be effective, there are details and safety rules that everyone should learn first. In this chapter, we will look at how castor oil works on the digestive system, the best ways to use it, and the possible risks that come with using too much or using it incorrectly. We will also discuss special considerations for certain groups, like pregnant people, the elderly, and those with ongoing health issues. By the end, you should have a balanced view of how castor oil can support the digestive system.

## 1. Overview of Castor Oil's Digestive Effects

When castor oil is swallowed, it can trigger the intestines to move more actively. This effect comes largely from ricinoleic acid, the main fatty acid in castor oil. Once castor oil reaches the small intestine, enzymes help break it down. That process releases substances that can prompt the muscle walls of the intestines to contract more. As a result, waste travels faster through the digestive tract, leading to a bowel movement.

This is why castor oil has been labeled a laxative. However, it is considered a strong laxative. While it might help with simple constipation in some cases, it is not mild. Swallowing a bit more than recommended can lead to cramping, diarrhea, or dehydration if a person is not careful. Because of this power, many doctors suggest more gentle laxatives first. But for those who still choose castor oil, knowing safe dosing guidelines is key.

## 2. Traditional Use for Occasional Constipation

Historically, families in various places have used castor oil to relieve constipation. Some grandparents might recall getting a spoonful of castor oil as children when they had trouble passing waste. This was often seen as a quick fix that could clear the bowels.

Yet, traditional use did not always include detailed measurements. Some folks used a tablespoon, others a teaspoon, and the results could vary widely. One person might find relief, while another might spend the day in the bathroom with cramps. Over time, health workers realized that it would be better to have more exact dosing instructions. They also learned that certain people (for example, pregnant people or those with certain conditions) should be very cautious with castor oil or avoid it altogether.

---

## 3. How to Measure a Dose

If you decide to use castor oil for occasional constipation, you need to measure it accurately. Generally, dosing guidelines mention anywhere from one teaspoon (about 5 milliliters) up to one tablespoon (about 15 milliliters) for adults. The actual amount depends on your body weight, how your body reacts, and advice from a reliable health source. Some people start with the smaller dose to test how it affects them. That is often a wise step.

It is best to check the product label or any leaflet that comes with the bottle. If there is no label, you can look at trustworthy references or speak with a pharmacist. It is also important to keep in mind that castor oil tastes strong and can be unpleasant. That is why some people mix it with juice or water. Still, the flavor and thickness can be noticeable no matter how you try to hide it.

---

## 4. Timing and Preparation

Timing matters when taking castor oil by mouth:

1. **Pick a Day Off:** Because castor oil can work quickly, it is wise to choose a time when you do not have to leave home. Some people feel the urge to go to the bathroom within 2-6 hours after taking it.
2. **Stay Hydrated:** Keep water nearby and sip regularly to help avoid dehydration, especially if you have multiple bowel movements.
3. **Mixing Options:** If you find the taste unpleasant, you can mix castor oil with a small glass of orange juice, lemon juice, or ginger tea. Others chill the oil in the fridge for a short time, which can slightly change the texture and taste.
4. **Avoid Large Meals Right Away:** Since castor oil may bring on bowel movements, you might not want to have a heavy meal immediately before or after. Light foods, soups, or broths may be easier on the stomach.

## 5. Potential Benefits When Used Carefully

1. **Clearing Occasional Backup:** For those dealing with short-term constipation, castor oil can help move things along.
2. **Reducing Temporary Discomfort:** If someone feels bloated or slightly unwell because of backed-up bowels, a proper dose might relieve that feeling.
3. **Long-Standing Tradition:** Because people have used it for a long time, some feel more comfortable with a natural oil than with modern laxatives. Though "natural" does not always mean safer, it can appeal to those who prefer plant-based products.

Still, castor oil is not a daily solution. Using it too often can make your bowels depend on it. Overuse might also bother the gut lining or lead to issues like electrolyte imbalances. Once again, caution is key.

## 6. Risks and Side Effects

Castor oil's strong laxative power means that side effects are possible. Here are the main things to watch:

1. **Stomach Cramps:** Because it forces the intestines to contract more than usual, cramping is common. This can be mild or quite uncomfortable.
2. **Diarrhea:** Taking more than recommended can lead to watery stools and frequent trips to the bathroom. This can cause dehydration, so it is wise to drink extra fluids.
3. **Nausea or Vomiting:** The thick taste and strong odor can cause some people to feel queasy.
4. **Dehydration:** Passing a large amount of waste in a short time can cause the body to lose fluids and electrolytes. That is why it is vital to replace lost fluids with water or clear drinks.
5. **Bowel Dependence:** Overusing any strong laxative may weaken the body's natural urge to pass waste. That can make constipation worse over time.

## 7. Special Warnings for Pregnant People

A common old tip is that pregnant people can use castor oil to "help labor start." However, this is not something to do without medical advice. Castor oil can bring on powerful contractions not only in the intestines but sometimes in the uterus. This could lead to early labor or stress for the baby. Many health workers do not suggest castor oil for pregnancy unless they are monitoring the patient closely.

If someone is expecting and has constipation, they should talk to a healthcare worker. There are gentler options that can be used during pregnancy. Using castor oil on your own can carry serious risks for both the parent and the baby.

## 8. Tips for Older Adults

Older adults may have more delicate systems, as well as chronic health issues or medicines that might mix poorly with castor oil's effects. Dehydration is also a bigger worry in this age group, since the body's thirst signals can be less reliable, and the kidneys might not handle sudden fluid loss as well. Because of these concerns:

1. **Start Small:** If castor oil is used, start at the lowest dose.
2. **Check Medications:** Some medicines can be disrupted by diarrhea or changes in electrolytes.
3. **Stay in Touch with a Health Professional:** Let them know you plan to use castor oil, so they can advise on safety steps.

For many older people, a mild stool softener or an increase in dietary fiber might be a safer route than castor oil.

---

## 9. Dos and Don'ts

**Dos:**

- **Do measure carefully.**
- **Do drink extra water.**
- **Do stay near a bathroom.**
- **Do talk to a professional if you have ongoing constipation.**

**Don'ts:**

- **Don't take castor oil often.** It is not meant for daily use.
- **Don't ignore severe cramping or ongoing diarrhea.** If these happen, consider getting medical help.
- **Don't mix castor oil with substances that might irritate the gut further.**
- **Don't rely on castor oil if you have a serious gut issue or unknown abdominal pain.**

---

## 10. Mixing Castor Oil with Herbs or Teas

Some people try mixing castor oil with herbal teas like ginger or peppermint to ease nausea or cramping. While this might help with taste and mild soothing, it is not guaranteed to remove all side effects. Others add castor oil to certain herbal blends that support digestion, hoping for a gentle effect. If you choose this path, make sure none of the herbs interacts badly with your body or your current medicines. Always use small amounts first to see how your body reacts.

## 11. Lesser-Known Tips (Additional Caution)

1. **Split Doses:** Instead of taking one larger dose, some prefer dividing it into two smaller doses a few hours apart. This can sometimes reduce intense cramps.
2. **Timing Before Bed:** Some folks think taking castor oil at night is easier, but it might disrupt sleep if the urge to go to the bathroom hits in the middle of the night.
3. **Watch for Signs of Overuse:** If you begin needing castor oil for every bowel movement, that is a red flag. It may mean your bowels are adjusting to the laxative, and you should seek advice.
4. **Check for Interactions:** If you are on medicines for blood pressure, diabetes, or other conditions, diarrhea can affect how your body handles those drugs. Keep an eye out for unusual symptoms.

## 12. When to Seek Professional Help

Castor oil is meant for short-term relief of mild constipation. If the problem is severe, or if you notice any of the following, it is time to seek help:

- **Blood in Stool:** This can indicate a serious condition.
- **Severe Abdominal Pain:** This might not be normal constipation and could be something else.
- **Long-Term Constipation:** If it keeps coming back or lasting for weeks, you need more investigation.
- **Signs of Severe Dehydration:** This includes extreme thirst, dizziness, or feeling faint.

Waiting too long to address these warning signs can make the situation worse, so it is always better to be cautious.

## 13. Children and Castor Oil

When it comes to children, castor oil is typically not advised unless a health professional specifically says so. Children's bodies are smaller and can dehydrate faster. A strong laxative might cause them severe discomfort or electrolyte problems. In many cases, more gentle methods are safer, like adding more fiber to their diet or using mild stool softeners that are designed for kids. If a child is severely constipated, a pediatrician should be involved in deciding the best treatment.

## 14. Myths Around Castor Oil for Digestion

1. **"More Oil Means Better Results":** This is wrong. Taking more than recommended can lead to too many trips to the bathroom or painful cramps.
2. **"Safe for Everyone Because It's Natural":** Even though it is a plant-based oil, castor oil can be risky if used incorrectly.
3. **"It Will Clear All Toxins":** Some people claim castor oil purges the body of toxins. While it can help clear waste, the body has its own detox systems (like the liver and kidneys). Castor oil does not clean out every "toxin" that might be in your body.

## 15. Longer-Term Gut Health

If you find yourself dealing with constipation often, relying on castor oil each time is not a good plan. Addressing the root causes can bring more relief in the long run. You might need to:

- **Increase Fiber Intake:** Whole grains, fruits, vegetables, and beans can support healthy bowel movements.
- **Drink More Fluids:** Water, herbal teas, and other clear drinks can help stools pass more easily.

- **Exercise Regularly:** Even simple walks can help keep the intestines moving.
- **Check Medications:** Some drugs can cause constipation. Ask your health worker if there are alternatives.
- **Evaluate Stress:** Stress can affect digestion. Methods such as slow breathing or short calming activities might help with bowel habits.

---

## 16. Rare But Possible Serious Problems

While most healthy adults who use a single small dose of castor oil will only experience the typical laxative effects, there are rare cases where castor oil caused more severe complications. For example, if someone is extremely dehydrated to begin with, losing more fluid through diarrhea can worsen that problem fast. Also, if a person has a gut blockage or certain inflammatory conditions, forcing the bowels to move could be dangerous.

This is why reading reliable sources and possibly speaking to a health professional is important before using castor oil for the first time, especially if you have any health problems or take medications regularly.

---

## 17. Combining Castor Oil Packs with Internal Use?

Some folks wonder if they should do a castor oil pack on the abdomen while also swallowing the oil to "enhance" the effect. That is usually not recommended. A castor oil pack on the abdomen is often aimed at comfort or mild external soothing. Swallowing the oil at the same time might double the stimulation of the intestines, which can be overwhelming. If you want to try both methods, speak to a professional, or at least do them at different times to see how your body handles each one.

## 18. Ideas for Gentle Alternatives

If you are not sure about castor oil or find it too strong, there are other gentle paths to support digestion:

1. **Prune Juice:** Many people use prune juice or dried prunes for mild constipation. Prunes have natural fiber and sorbitol, which can help the bowels.
2. **Psyllium Husk:** This is a soluble fiber that can be mixed with water or juice to help form softer, bulkier stools.
3. **Magnesium Supplements:** Certain forms of magnesium act as mild laxatives by drawing water into the intestines.
4. **Herbal Teas:** Senna tea or smooth move tea might help but can also cause cramps. They are still often milder than castor oil.
5. **Diet and Activity Changes:** As noted earlier, focusing on fiber, water, and moderate exercise can go a long way.

---

## 19. Real-World Examples (Without Personal Names)

- **Case A:** A middle-aged office worker tried a tablespoon of castor oil on a weekend after feeling blocked for three days. Within four hours, he had a bowel movement. He felt relief, but he also had to visit the bathroom several times. He decided to look into more fiber-rich foods to prevent repeated use.
- **Case B:** An older person with heart medicine took castor oil to help with constipation. She became dizzy and realized her blood pressure medicine was not working the same, possibly due to fluid loss and electrolyte changes. She then spoke with a doctor and switched to a gentler approach.

These examples show that while castor oil can help, it can also come with downsides. Everyone's body reacts differently.

---

## 20. Step-by-Step Safe Use Plan

If you have chosen to try castor oil for a one-time constipation episode:

1. **Confirm It's Right for You:** Do not have any major health condition or take medicines that could be affected by diarrhea.
2. **Plan a Clear Day:** Make sure you can stay at home and do not have pressing errands.
3. **Start Low:** Try 1 teaspoon instead of a full tablespoon.
4. **Mix with a Pleasant Drink:** For example, orange juice.
5. **Wait and See:** Give it at least 4 hours to work. Do not take an extra dose too soon.
6. **Drink Water:** Aim for a glass of water every hour or two.
7. **Monitor Body Reactions:** If cramps are severe or if you feel dizzy, consider calling a professional.
8. **Limit Use to One Time:** Avoid repeating doses over the next days unless a health worker says otherwise.

---

## 21. Checking the Quality of the Oil

Although castor oil sold in pharmacies for internal use should meet certain standards, you might still want to check the label. Make sure it is labeled for internal use or "food-grade." Some castor oils on the market are only for external uses (like cosmetic or hair care) and might contain added ingredients not meant to be swallowed. Look for purity statements. If unsure, ask the store staff or look for a brand you trust.

---

## 22. Handling Side Effects at Home

If you feel mild cramps or slight nausea after a proper dose of castor oil:

- **Try Gentle Belly Rubs:** Sometimes softly rubbing the abdomen can ease muscle spasms.
- **Warm Compress:** Placing a warm towel or a mild heating pad on the abdomen can offer comfort. Make sure not to burn the skin.

- **Light Diet:** Eat easy-to-digest foods like toast or bananas if you feel a little shaky.
- **Replenish Electrolytes:** If you have had a lot of diarrhea, a clear broth or an oral rehydration drink might help replace lost electrolytes.

If the cramping or nausea gets worse or you see any red-flag signs, seek help.

---

## 23. Can Castor Oil Help with Bloating?

Some people do not have true constipation but struggle with bloating. Castor oil might move things along, but if bloating is not caused by being backed up, castor oil will not solve the underlying cause. Bloating can be related to food sensitivities, slow digestion, or gut bacteria imbalances. It might be wise to track what triggers your bloating, see if there are certain foods that worsen it, and try to address it in a more focused way.

---

## 24. Mindset About Using Laxatives

Using laxatives should be a last resort for occasional problems, not a normal part of daily life. The gut is designed to function on its own. Overuse of laxatives can weaken that natural function or hide signs of a deeper issue. If you are constantly turning to castor oil or other laxatives, it might be time to speak with a health worker and get to the root of your digestive issues.

# CHAPTER 8: IMMUNE SYSTEM EFFECTS

Castor oil has been linked to several ideas about how it might help the body beyond just aiding the bowels or softening the skin. One interesting point is whether castor oil can affect the immune system. Some people believe that using castor oil packs on the abdomen or joints helps the body fight off minor issues and supports overall health. Others talk about how ricinoleic acid might play a role in reducing minor swelling that can be tied to immune responses. In this chapter, we will explore these claims, look at current knowledge, and see what steps you can take if you hope to use castor oil as part of a natural approach to basic immune support. Remember that serious immune problems should be handled by professional care. Still, for those wanting a simple home method, there may be some points of interest here.

## 1. Basic Understanding of the Immune System

The immune system is the body's defense network. It identifies foreign substances like bacteria and viruses, then acts to remove or neutralize them. In addition, the immune system is involved in recognizing and handling damaged or old cells in the body. When the immune system is balanced, a person can respond well to common pathogens and heal from small wounds. When it is out of balance, issues can arise, such as frequent colds or slower recovery from minor infections.

Many factors influence immune health. A balanced diet, regular movement, good sleep, and effective stress management play key roles. While natural products like castor oil might support certain aspects, it is important to see them as part of a bigger picture. Castor oil alone is not a cure-all for serious immune deficiencies or conditions.

## 2. The Idea Behind Castor Oil Packs

A castor oil pack is a piece of cloth soaked in castor oil, placed on the skin (often on the abdomen), and kept warm with a heating pad or hot water bottle. Some say this method supports lymph flow and helps the body clear waste more efficiently. The lymphatic system is part of the immune network. It carries lymph fluid, which includes white blood cells that fight infection.

Fans of this method claim that castor oil packs might gently encourage better circulation in the area underneath the cloth. If blood flow and lymph movement improve, the body could handle minor invaders more quickly. However, solid scientific evidence on these claims is limited. Most of the support comes from personal experiences and small studies rather than large-scale clinical trials.

---

## 3. Possible Effects of Ricinoleic Acid on Minor Swelling

Ricinoleic acid is often linked to reducing minor swelling when applied to the skin. In certain lab tests, this fatty acid slowed down some of the signals that cause cells to become puffy and irritated. While these findings are interesting, they do not necessarily prove that rubbing castor oil on your body can block large-scale immune problems. That said, for mild aches or areas that feel a bit inflamed, some people find relief using warm castor oil rubs. It might soothe the area, offering short-term comfort.

---

## 4. Supporting Skin as an Immune Barrier

One of the first lines of immune defense is the skin itself. When the skin is intact, it blocks many germs from entering the body. Castor oil may help keep the skin moisturized and less prone to cracks. If your hands, feet, or other areas of skin stay soft and free from splits, you reduce possible entry points for bacteria.

In a minor sense, by helping the skin remain healthy, castor oil might support part of your immune defense. This does not mean castor oil kills all germs or replaces normal cleanliness. It just means well-moisturized skin can do its job of defense more effectively than dry, cracked skin.

## 5. Warm Compresses and Comfort

When you apply a warm compress or castor oil pack, you might feel relaxed. Stress can weaken the immune system if it becomes chronic. By taking a short time to lie down with a gentle warmth on the abdomen or back, you might reduce tension levels. If your stress is lower, your immune response might indirectly benefit. This is an indirect effect rather than a direct chemical action of the oil. Still, it shows how a calming routine can help overall well-being.

## 6. Minor Joint Aches and Immune Connections

Some minor joint aches might be tied to basic wear and tear, while others might relate to immune responses that cause inflammation in the joints. While castor oil is not a proven treatment for major joint conditions, some people report that rubbing warm castor oil on sore joints can reduce discomfort for a short time. This is likely because the oil soothes the skin and keeps the area warm, rather than making a deep immune change. However, if a joint feels less stiff, you might move more easily, helping with blood flow and possibly giving small benefits to the immune system's normal cleanup tasks.

## 7. Digestive Health and Immunity

A large part of the immune system is located in the gut. The health of the gut lining and the balance of gut microbes can influence how the immune system reacts to everyday challenges. If you occasionally use castor oil to help with constipation (as mentioned in the previous chapter), you might keep your digestive system running more smoothly. In theory, less backup in the intestines could mean fewer toxins or irritants sitting in the gut. This does not guarantee a massive boost to immune power, but a healthier gut may help you feel better overall.

That said, taking castor oil too often can be rough on your system. Frequent diarrhea or cramping might disturb gut balance, leading to other issues. As with many things, moderation is crucial.

---

## 8. Possible Role in Basic Detox Routines

Some health seekers talk about "detox," meaning ways to help the body remove what they consider harmful substances. The body naturally clears waste through the liver, kidneys, lungs, and skin. Castor oil is sometimes included in home "cleanse" routines, either by swallowing a measured dose or by using packs. The idea is that castor oil may speed up the removal of old waste in the bowels, or that a pack might support the liver area when placed on the right side of the abdomen.

However, medical research does not strongly confirm that castor oil has a big effect on the liver's detox function. The best approach to supporting the liver is to avoid too much alcohol, eat a balanced diet, and stay hydrated. Castor oil might help with mild constipation or offer a warm, soothing effect on the abdomen, but claiming it alone can "clean out" all toxins is not supported by strong evidence.

---

## 9. Caring for Lymph Nodes Externally?

Some individuals apply castor oil to areas where lymph nodes are located, such as behind the knees, in the armpits, or along the neck. They believe that this can help the lymphatic system move fluid. While a gentle massage with any oil could help the local flow of fluids, whether castor oil itself has a special effect is open to question. There is no firm scientific proof that castor oil can dramatically change lymph function. However, the warmth and massaging motion might make the area feel less tight, which can be comforting.

## 10. Avoiding Overclaims and Looking for Balance

Many claims about castor oil and the immune system can be found online. Some are reasonable, while others are quite extreme. It is important to keep expectations realistic. If someone has a serious immune disorder, castor oil is not likely to fix it. If you have a mild issue, like a small patch of inflamed skin, a bit of castor oil might bring some relief. That relief could give the immune system one less irritation to manage, but it does not mean castor oil is a full immune booster by itself.

## 11. Simple Methods to Try at Home

1. **Warm Abdomen Pack:** Warm a piece of cotton cloth soaked in castor oil, place it on your abdomen, and cover with plastic wrap. Add a heating pad on low, and rest for about 30 minutes. This might help you feel calm and possibly support gentle circulation in the area.
2. **Joint Comfort Rub:** Mix a few drops of castor oil with a lighter oil, warm it slightly, then massage it into mildly achy joints. Do not expect a cure, but the warmth and moisture could ease some tension.
3. **Neck or Underarm Gentle Massage:** If you feel tightness around the neck or armpits, a gentle self-massage with castor oil may relax those areas. Keep pressure light and stop if you feel pain.

## 12. Signs of a Balanced Immune Response

While using castor oil packs or rubs, you might wonder if it is having any effect on your immune system at all. Some signs of a healthy immune response include:

- **Regular Energy Levels:** You do not feel worn out all the time.
- **Normal Recovery:** Small cuts or colds heal in a usual time frame.
- **No Ongoing Redness or Swelling:** Skin issues are mild and go away quickly.
- **Digestive Comfort:** You do not frequently experience severe bloating or irregular bowel movements.

If you notice that you feel more relaxed, sleep better, or have fewer mild aches, that could be related to using castor oil as part of a calming routine. Or it might just be that you are taking better care of yourself overall.

---

## 13. The Importance of Whole-Body Health

It can be tempting to focus on one product like castor oil and forget the rest of your lifestyle. But building strong defenses usually involves:

1. **Eating Nutrient-Rich Foods:** Fruits, vegetables, lean proteins, and healthy fats supply vitamins and minerals that support immune cells.
2. **Staying Active:** Regular walks or other forms of movement can boost circulation, which in turn can help the immune cells move through the body more effectively.
3. **Getting Enough Sleep:** Sleep is when the body repairs tissues and organizes immune responses.
4. **Managing Stress:** Chronic stress can interfere with healthy immune function.
5. **Staying Hydrated:** Water helps transport nutrients to cells and carry waste away.

Castor oil might be a small part of your plan, but it is no substitute for these larger pieces.

## 14. Studies and Observations (What We Know So Far)

Large-scale studies on castor oil and direct immune effects are limited. Some smaller studies or anecdotal reports suggest benefits for minor inflammation or stress-related aches. Others note that castor oil packs can improve comfort in some individuals, leading to better rest. However, these findings are not enough to say castor oil is a proven immune booster.

Researchers sometimes focus on ricinoleic acid and how it interacts with certain enzymes in the body that influence swelling or tissue response. This research is ongoing. If future studies shed more light, we might have a clearer explanation of when and how castor oil can help with immune-related concerns. For now, it is mainly a matter of personal choice, guided by basic safety.

---

## 15. Could Ricin in the Seeds Affect the Immune System?

Ricin, the harmful protein in raw castor seeds, is removed or destroyed during proper oil processing. It is known to be toxic in its raw form. But in purified castor oil, there should be no harmful level of ricin. Therefore, you do not need to worry about ricin poisoning if you purchase from a reliable brand that follows proper steps. The immune effects sometimes linked to ricin have nothing to do with safe castor oil used at home.

---

## 16. Combining Castor Oil with Other Immune-Friendly Items

Some people try to boost the soothing effects of a castor oil pack by adding a few drops of mild essential oils that are thought to support overall comfort, like chamomile or frankincense. If you use essential oils, be sure they are safe for topical use. Also do a patch test, as essential oils can cause reactions in some people. The combination may feel pleasant and relaxing, which might help calm the body. But again, these methods should not replace professional care if you have a serious condition.

## 17. Using Castor Oil During Mild Seasonal Changes

When seasons shift, some individuals feel more tired or catch mild illnesses. A warm castor oil pack on the abdomen or chest might offer comfort. Some families pass down a practice of placing a small castor oil pack on the chest with gentle heat to ease mild congestion, although there is no solid proof it solves respiratory problems. Still, the warmth might help you relax, which can support your body's natural responses.

## 18. Watching for Any Sensitivities

If you notice more redness or irritation after using castor oil packs, you might be sensitive to either castor oil itself or the heat. Remove the pack and wash the area. If the irritation persists, do not continue this approach. Some people find that they do better with shorter pack sessions, like 15-20 minutes instead of an hour. Also, ensure the oil is not too hot when you apply it, as you do not want to scald the skin.

## 19. Simple Checklist for Castor Oil Immune Support

1. **Pick Quality Oil:** Make sure the oil is clean, pure, and safe for skin application.
2. **Warm Gently:** Avoid high heat that could degrade the oil or burn you.
3. **Test a Small Area:** Before placing a pack on a large area, test a tiny patch of skin to see if there is a reaction.
4. **Relax:** Use the time you have the pack on to rest, do slow breathing, or even listen to calming music.
5. **Observe Changes:** Notice if you feel less stiffness or mild improvement in well-being, but keep realistic expectations.
6. **Maintain a Healthy Routine:** Do not drop your other good habits or any medical treatment you are already on.

## 20. Could Castor Oil Help with Mild Headaches?

Some mild headaches are linked to tension in the muscles or the base of the neck. Rubbing a bit of castor oil on the neck or temples might ease tightness. The warmth from gentle massage can help release muscle tension, which might lessen certain headache symptoms. This is more related to relaxation than a direct immune effect, but being pain-free could reduce stress on the body's defenses.

## 21. Supporting the Body After a Cold

Once you have gotten over a cold or mild illness, your body is in recovery mode. Some people think a castor oil pack on the abdomen or lower back helps them feel comforted, giving them a chance to rest more deeply. If you believe it helps, it can be included in a wider plan of recovery: good nutrition, enough fluids, and gradual return to normal activities. Keep in mind that if you are still feeling weak or have lingering symptoms, you should consider a professional check-up.

## 22. Myths and Overstatements

1. **"Castor Oil Can Fix All Immune Problems"**: Not true. Major immune problems need specialized care.
2. **"No Risk of Overuse"**: Using castor oil on the skin too often or in large amounts could cause irritation or mess with your daily routine.
3. **"Swallowing More Castor Oil Boosts the Immune System"**: Taking extra internally can lead to digestive upset and dehydration. It is not a good way to seek better immune function.

## 23. Handling More Serious Inflammation

If someone is dealing with a health condition that involves chronic or serious inflammation, such as autoimmune disorders, they need proper medical guidance. Castor oil might be a side method to soothe skin or help reduce mild aches, but it cannot replace medicines or treatments that control serious flare-ups. Always talk to a health worker before adding new methods to your plan, especially if you already take medicines that affect the immune system.

---

## 24. Listening to Your Body's Signals

When trying castor oil for mild immune-related support, pay attention to how your body reacts:

- **Immediate Discomfort:** Stop if you feel odd or if pain increases.
- **Positive Relaxation:** If you feel calmer and notice less minor swelling, that might be a sign the method is okay for you.
- **Changes Over Time:** If you see no difference after several tries, you may not be someone who benefits from castor oil packs in this way.

Everyone's body is unique, so do not force something that seems unhelpful or that causes trouble.

# CHAPTER 9: LIVER AND ORGAN HEALTH

Castor oil is often linked to external uses like skin and hair care, but there are also folks who point to a possible link between castor oil and organ health, especially the liver. The liver is a key organ. It helps filter unwanted materials from the blood, manages nutrients, and carries out many roles that keep the body balanced. In this chapter, we will look at how some people apply castor oil packs over the liver or other parts of the abdomen, hoping to support basic organ health. We will look at traditional ideas and modern thoughts, along with tips and caution points. While some reports sound promising, keep in mind that if you have serious organ or liver concerns, you should look for professional help.

## 1. Why the Liver Matters

The liver sits under the right side of the rib cage. It is large, spongy, and vital for many tasks:

- It filters out some unwanted substances.
- It helps change nutrients from our food into usable forms.
- It makes and secretes bile, which helps break down fats.
- It stores certain vitamins and sugar (in the form of glycogen).

If the liver is strained or not working well, a person might feel tired or have digestive troubles. In serious cases, toxins can build up in the blood. To keep the liver strong, many people focus on a good diet, limiting heavy alcohol use, and staying hydrated. Castor oil packs are a side method that some try for general help.

## 2. What People Claim About Castor Oil and the Liver

Some alternative health practices say that putting a castor oil pack on the right side of the abdomen (over the liver area) might:

- Help with blood flow to that region.
- Support the body's normal "clean-up" actions.
- Ease mild discomfort in the abdomen.
- Make a person feel calmer, which might have indirect benefits for organ function.

Although there are not big scientific trials proving these points, personal stories are common. People say things like, "I felt less bloated," or "My digestion seemed smoother after a week of doing castor oil packs." These are personal accounts rather than data from large studies.

---

## 3. How a Castor Oil Pack for the Liver Is Often Done

1. **Choose Your Cloth:** Many people use a piece of wool flannel or cotton. The cloth should be thick enough to hold a good amount of oil but not so thick that it will not bend around your body.
2. **Warm the Oil:** Warm a small amount of castor oil by placing the bottle in a bowl of warm water. It should feel comfortably warm, not hot.
3. **Soak the Cloth:** Pour enough castor oil on the cloth so that it is well-saturated but not dripping.
4. **Apply to Your Right Side:** Lie down or recline in a way that you can place the cloth over the liver area, which is generally the upper right side of the abdomen.
5. **Cover It:** Some folks wrap plastic over the cloth to keep the oil from making a mess. Others use an old towel.
6. **Add Heat (Optional):** Place a heating pad or hot water bottle on top of the cloth if you want gentle warmth.
7. **Relax for 30 to 60 Minutes:** Use this time to stay still, read a book, or rest.
8. **Clean Up:** When you are finished, remove the cloth and wipe away extra oil with a paper towel or a damp cloth.

Some do this practice a few times a week, maybe before bed. They claim it helps them rest better or that they feel a calmness in the abdomen.

---

## 4. What Does Science Say?

There are not many large-scale, peer-reviewed studies on castor oil packs and the liver. Some small studies suggest that castor oil packs can help reduce mild constipation or occasional swelling. But when it comes to direct, proven effects on the liver's filtering tasks, we do not have strong scientific evidence. That does not mean it does nothing. It just means we do not yet have clear proof that a warm castor oil pack can change deep organ activity in a big way.

Because castor oil has a unique fatty acid (ricinoleic acid), some researchers have looked at how it might reduce certain irritations or calm tissues. It is possible that the gentle warmth and moisture on the skin also boost local blood flow. Better blood flow might help the body's normal processes. Still, this remains a theory without large human trials.

---

## 5. Can Castor Oil Packs Replace Medical Treatments?

No. If someone has a known liver condition such as hepatitis, cirrhosis, or a high level of liver enzymes on lab tests, castor oil packs are not a medical treatment. They might be a gentle practice you can do alongside the guidance of a professional, but they cannot fix the underlying condition. The same is true for kidney or pancreas issues. If you have organ trouble, you need specialized care.

Castor oil packs are generally seen as a home approach. They might add comfort or a sense of relaxation. Some folks believe it helps them avoid mild congestion in the abdomen area. But do not stop medications or other treatments just because you are doing a home method. Always speak with a health worker about changes in your care plan.

# 6. Using Castor Oil for Other Organs: Stomach, Kidneys, and More

While the liver area is the most common site for castor oil packs, some apply them to other parts of the abdomen:

- **Over the stomach:** in hopes of calming mild digestive upset.
- **Over the lower abdomen:** to ease light cramps.
- **Over the kidneys:** though this is less common.

Regardless of location, the method is similar: soak a cloth, place it on the target area, add gentle heat if desired, and rest. Some folks say they place the pack for about 30 minutes a few times a week to keep the region comfortable. Again, strong data is not there, but anecdotal reports continue to spread.

---

# 7. Possible Reasons People Feel Better

If someone says they feel less stomach pain or less abdominal tightness after a series of castor oil packs, what might be happening?

1. **Warmth Helps Muscles Relax:** Heat by itself can reduce muscle tension.
2. **Oil Soothes the Skin:** The thick castor oil might keep the skin warm and moist, promoting a calming effect.
3. **Quiet Time to Rest:** Spending half an hour lying down is a break from the day's stress, which can help the body settle.
4. **Mild Lymph Flow Support:** Some believe that the gentle heat and slight pressure can help the lymphatic system move fluids.

Each of these factors may bring a sense of relief, even if it is not a direct "cleansing" of the liver or other organs.

## 8. Avoiding Common Mistakes

1. **Overheating the Oil:** Do not microwave castor oil or heat it until it is scalding. Too much heat might hurt your skin.
2. **Leaving the Pack on Too Long:** Most people say 30-60 minutes is enough. Leaving it on all night could cause irritation, stains, or dryness.
3. **Skipping the Clean-Up:** Castor oil is thick. If you do not wipe it off well, it might rub on clothes or bedding.
4. **Expecting Instant Medical Cures:** Using a castor oil pack once or twice will not fix major conditions. It might bring mild comfort at best.
5. **Using Old or Unclean Cloths:** Always use fresh or well-washed materials to reduce the chance of skin irritation or bacterial growth.

---

## 9. Could Castor Oil Packs Stress the Liver?

Some individuals worry that if castor oil triggers the bowels or changes circulation, it could "stress" the liver. In most healthy adults, an occasional castor oil pack should not harm the liver. The method is external, and most of the oil's action stays on the surface of the skin. Unless you are swallowing the oil in large amounts, there is no heavy load on the liver. Of course, if you have a rare sensitivity or open sores on your abdomen, you should talk to a health professional.

---

## 10. Thoughts on "Detox" Language

You might see some writings that say castor oil "detoxifies" the liver. The term "detox" can be confusing. The body is designed to handle waste through the liver, kidneys, and other systems. A warm castor oil pack might help you relax, which can support overall health. However, it is not correct to say that castor oil alone washes out toxins on a grand scale. The best ways to keep your liver happy are:

- Limiting harmful substances like heavy alcohol or too many processed foods.
- Staying well-hydrated.
- Eating a balanced diet that has fruits, vegetables, and whole grains.
- Staying active.

Castor oil packs can be a small piece of a better routine, but they are not a free pass to ignore other healthy habits.

---

## 11. Tips for Gentle Support of Organs

Apart from castor oil, consider these ways to look after your liver and other organs:

1. **Stay Hydrated:** Water helps your organs flush out waste.
2. **Eat Enough Fiber:** Vegetables, beans, and whole grains can help the bowels move and reduce strain on the liver.
3. **Avoid Binge Drinking:** Alcohol can damage liver cells. If you do drink, keep it moderate.
4. **Check Medicines:** Some medicines can stress the liver if misused. Follow directions.
5. **Use Castor Oil in Moderation:** If you enjoy castor oil packs, do them responsibly.

---

## 12. Personal Schedules and Daily Routines

Some individuals add castor oil packs into a weekly or monthly regimen. For example:

- **Twice a Week:** They might place a castor oil pack over the liver area on Tuesday and Thursday evenings, letting it sit for 30 minutes each time.
- **Monthly Routine:** Others do a short "wellness day" once a month, where they rest, drink plenty of water, eat light meals, and apply a castor oil pack while reading.

These gentle habits can help a person slow down and pay attention to how they feel. This break from busy life might be the biggest advantage of using a pack.

## 13. Watching for Skin Reactions

Your abdomen may not be used to thick oil for extended periods. Watch for:

- **Rashes** or small bumps.
- **Redness** that remains after you remove the pack.
- **Itchiness** under the cloth.

If these appear, reduce how long you leave the pack on. Check if you are using too much heat or if you have an allergy to the cloth material. Some folks switch to a lighter oil mix (like half castor oil, half another oil) if pure castor oil is too thick on the skin.

## 14. Using Castor Oil on the Sides of the Abdomen or Back

The human body has more organs in the abdominal region than just the liver. Some folks like to place castor oil packs on the left side for the spleen area or near the lower back for the kidneys. The approach is the same. They hope the gentle warmth can relax tight muscles or ease mild soreness. While there is no large study proving big changes, the warming effect could offer comfort.

## 15. Fitting Castor Oil Into a Healthy Lifestyle

If you think of your health as a table supported by different legs (diet, exercise, sleep, and stress management), you might consider castor oil packs as an extra small support. It might help you rest or give you some sense of well-being, but it cannot stand alone to keep you healthy. Pair it with:

- **Enough Sleep:** Let your body recover each night.
- **Balanced Meals:** Focus on nutrients, not just calories.
- **Regular Movement:** Even short walks can help blood flow.
- **Stress Reduction:** Activities that calm the mind, such as mild stretches or easy breathing.

In that context, castor oil packs might add a gentle bonus.

## 16. Can Castor Oil Packs Help the Gallbladder?

The gallbladder, which sits under the liver, stores and releases bile to aid in fat digestion. Some alternative health sources say castor oil packs might help reduce mild gallbladder discomfort. If you have serious gallbladder issues like stones or inflammation, though, you need medical help. A warm pack might reduce mild cramping, but it does not break up real gallstones or treat infections. So do not rely on it for severe pain or if you suspect a major gallbladder concern.

## 17. Avoiding Overuse

If you find yourself wanting to do castor oil packs daily for hours at a time, take a step back. Overdoing any remedy can lead to new problems:

- Skin dryness or irritation.
- Extra cost and time without a clear benefit.
- A sense of false security, ignoring real medical advice.

Occasional use (like 2-3 times a week or less) is more balanced. If you see no benefit after a few weeks, it may not be the right approach for you.

## 18. Myths About "Melting Fat" or "Shrinking the Liver"

Some questionable sources claim that a castor oil pack can melt belly fat or shrink an enlarged liver. There is no proof for these ideas. Castor oil does not dissolve fat cells through the skin. If the liver is swollen due to disease, it needs proper care from a professional. It is better to focus on actual ways that castor oil can help, like mild relaxation or minor support for the skin and local circulation, instead of big unproven promises.

---

## 19. Trying a Castor Oil Blend for the Abdomen

If pure castor oil feels too thick or sticky, you can mix it with a lighter oil. For instance:

- **1 part castor oil**
- **1 part coconut oil** (or another mild oil)

Warm this blend, then apply it to the cloth. The mix might spread more evenly and still give you a comfortable, warm feeling. A ratio of 50:50 might be a good start. You can adjust as you see fit, maybe going 75% castor oil if you want a thicker mix.

---

## 20. Supporting the Liver With Food and Drink

While castor oil packs are external, the liver's main interactions come from what you eat and drink:

- **Leafy Greens:** Spinach, kale, and collards have nutrients that can help the body.
- **Cruciferous Veggies:** Broccoli, cauliflower, and cabbage contain elements that may support normal liver enzyme actions.
- **Green Tea or Herbal Teas:** Some people enjoy teas with mild antioxidants.
- **Beets and Berries:** These may help with normal inflammation levels.

If you already have a balanced diet, a castor oil pack is simply an extra comfort measure.

## 21. Using Gentle Pressure While Applying Castor Oil

Some folks choose to do a light massage before or after placing the castor oil cloth. This might help the abdominal muscles relax:

1. Warm your hands.
2. Put a small amount of castor oil on your fingertips.
3. Use slow, circular motions on the abdomen.
4. Be gentle—pushing too hard can be uncomfortable.
5. Then place the pack on top for the stated time.

This short massage could help with mild tension and might put you in a calmer state. Remember not to press too hard if you have pain or any known abdominal issue.

## 22. Keeping a Notebook

If you are curious about how castor oil packs might be helping you, keep a simple log. Write down:

- The day and time you applied the pack.
- How long you left it on.
- What you felt before, during, and after (e.g., relaxed, mild warmth, or nothing special).
- Any changes in digestion or discomfort.

After a few weeks, look for patterns. You might find that it helps you unwind or that you do not see much change. This record can guide you in deciding whether to keep using it.

## 23. Special Considerations for People With Certain Conditions

- **Pregnancy:** As mentioned in past chapters, pregnant individuals should be cautious with castor oil, especially swallowing it. For external use on the abdomen, some choose to avoid it entirely unless their health worker says it is okay.
- **Post-Surgery:** If you have had abdominal surgery, placing thick oil and heat on the area might not be advised until you heal. Always check with your care team.
- **Serious Liver Disease:** Speak to a doctor. A castor oil pack will not fix severe disease, and you need real medical treatment.
- **Open Wounds or Rashes:** Do not place castor oil packs over broken skin unless guided by a professional.

---

## 24. The Role of Attitude and Calmness

We cannot discount the effect of a calm mind on how we feel physically. If applying a warm castor oil pack on your abdomen encourages you to rest, breathe slowly, and turn off distractions for half an hour, that alone might help your body's overall state. Some who use these packs regularly say the biggest benefit is stress relief, which can have positive effects on various organs indirectly.

# CHAPTER 10: STRESS AND SLEEP SUPPORT

Many people today report high levels of stress. Jobs, family tasks, busy schedules, and a constant stream of news can weigh on the mind and body. In looking for ways to ease tension, some turn to natural products like castor oil. Although it might sound odd at first, there are reasons why castor oil could play a part in helping you calm down and prepare for better rest. From simple foot rubs to warm abdominal packs, a few of these methods might help soothe the body. In this chapter, we will go over how castor oil might help reduce stress levels and support more restful sleep, along with other tips you can combine it with.

## 1. The Link Between Relaxation and Castor Oil

Why would castor oil help a person feel calmer? The answer might lie in a few of its qualities:

1. **Thick Texture:** When rubbed on the skin, it can create a slow, deliberate sensation as you massage an area. This mindful act might help slow racing thoughts.
2. **Warmth and Comfort:** If used with a mild heating method, such as a castor oil pack or a warm foot bath, it can give a cozy feeling that signals the body to relax.
3. **Routine and Habit:** Setting aside time in the day to apply castor oil, even for just 10-15 minutes, can become part of a bedtime routine, telling your mind that it is time to wind down.

Though these points are not official medical therapy, they can be part of an overall approach to stress relief.

## 2. Common Stress-Related Habits

Before we move into specific castor oil methods, it helps to note a few daily habits that can build or reduce stress. Things like poor sleep, lack of breaks, and constant mental strain often keep our muscles and minds on edge. The result can be tension headaches, tight shoulders, or troubled sleep. Many people do not realize how daily stress can sneak up until it feels overwhelming.

Adding small self-care steps, such as a castor oil foot massage before bed, might be a chance to pause and notice how you feel. This short break can let you slow down your breathing, reflect on the day, and let go of worries. A small routine can have a bigger impact than you might guess.

## 3. How Stress Affects Sleep

When stress is not handled, it often messes up sleep. You might lie in bed with your mind racing. Or you might fall asleep but wake up feeling tense. Over time, poor sleep can raise stress further, creating a cycle that is hard to break. People look for solutions, sometimes turning to sleeping pills or other aids. While those have their place, many also seek gentle methods first, like warm baths, herbal teas, or natural oils.

## 4. Foot Rub with Castor Oil for Stress Relief

A quick and simple approach is to rub a small amount of castor oil into your feet. Here is a brief method:

1. **Wash and Dry Your Feet:** This removes dirt and warms them up if you use warm water.
2. **Sit Comfortably:** Find a chair or a spot on the couch where you can reach your feet easily.
3. **Use a Small Amount of Oil:** Castor oil is thick, so start with a pea-sized drop. You can always add more if needed.

4. **Gentle Massage:** Use circular motions on the soles, heels, and between the toes. Spend at least a minute or two on each foot.
5. **Focus on Breathing:** Inhale slowly as you press, exhale as you release. This can help your mind settle.
6. **Put on Socks (Optional):** Some people slip on cotton socks to keep the oil off the floor. This also helps lock in warmth.

This short foot care session can help you feel more at ease, especially if you do it close to bedtime. The combination of touch, mild pressure, and the smooth oil can signal the brain to let go of worries.

---

## 5. Castor Oil Pack for Stress and Sleep

Beyond foot rubs, castor oil packs might help you calm down. In Chapter 9, we looked at applying a castor oil pack over the liver area for organ support, but you can place a pack on the lower abdomen or even on the chest if that feels more comfortable.

**Why It May Help:**

- The slight pressure of the pack and the warmth can relax abdominal or chest muscles.
- Lying still for 20-30 minutes is a chance to practice slower breathing or simply rest without gadgets.
- Some folks say it helps them feel "less on edge," which could be enough to ease the shift into sleep mode.

---

## 6. A Pre-Bed Routine Using Castor Oil

If you are a person who struggles with nighttime stress, consider creating a short ritual:

1. **Dim Lights:** About 30 minutes before bed, start lowering the brightness in your room or turn off overhead lights.
2. **Phone-Free Time:** Put your phone away or set it to "silent."

3. **Apply Castor Oil:** You could do a quick foot rub or place a castor oil pack on the abdomen.
4. **Quiet Activity:** While the oil pack sits, you might do a calm pastime like reading a light book (not a thriller), listening to gentle music, or just resting with your eyes closed.
5. **Clean Up and Go to Bed:** Remove the pack, wipe off extra oil if needed, and slip into bed.

Sticking to this routine can help train your brain to know that when these steps start, it is time to slow down.

---

## 7. Castor Oil and Tense Muscles

Stress often shows up as tight muscles in the neck, shoulders, or back. You might try a small castor oil massage on these spots, though it can be tricky to reach certain areas on your own. If you have someone to help you, or if you can reach your neck and shoulders, you can warm a small amount of castor oil and gently rub tight areas:

- **Keep Pressure Mild:** Pressing too hard might cause soreness.
- **Short Session:** Even 5 minutes can loosen mild tension.
- **Warm Compress:** After the massage, place a warm towel over the area for extra comfort.

This can be done any time you feel tension building, but many find it more effective before bed so they do not carry that stiffness into sleep.

---

## 8. Avoiding Over-Stimulation

If your stress is high, you might be tempted to watch TV or scroll on your phone to distract yourself. But bright screens and rapid content can keep your mind active. Instead, a slow, mindful act like rubbing castor oil on your feet or applying a warm pack might help shift your focus inward. In doing so, you might notice your breathing and let go of some tension. This calm approach could support better rest than falling asleep to loud or bright stimuli.

## 9. Adding Mild Scents (With Caution)

Some people like to mix a drop of a soothing essential oil (like lavender) with castor oil for a calming scent. If you decide to do this, be sure you:

- Use a skin-friendly essential oil.
- Test on a small patch of skin first to ensure you do not react.
- Use only 1-2 drops of essential oil per tablespoon of castor oil, as essential oils can be strong.

The mild scent might add a layer of relaxation. However, if you are sensitive to smells, it is fine to use plain castor oil.

---

## 10. Stress-Related Headaches and Castor Oil

Tense muscles in the head, neck, or jaw can trigger headaches. While castor oil is not a cure for migraines, a gentle massage on the temples or neck could help with mild tension headaches:

1. **Place a Little Castor Oil on Your Fingertips:** Warm it up by rubbing your hands together.
2. **Circle Motions on Temples:** Move in small circles, applying light pressure.
3. **Massage Behind Ears and Down the Neck:** This can help ease tight muscles that pull on the scalp.
4. **Avoid Getting Oil in the Hair:** Unless you are fine with washing your hair afterward, be careful around the hairline.

If the headache persists or worsens, it might be more than simple tension, and you could consider other remedies or speak with a professional.

---

## 11. Could Castor Oil Help with Anxiety?

Anxiety is a more complex state than everyday stress, often involving worry or panic feelings. While castor oil is not a medical treatment for anxiety, certain steps that accompany castor oil usage (such as calm breathing, gentle self-massage, or quiet time) can help a person manage mild anxious moments. If you have moderate or severe anxiety, it is best to get help from a mental health professional. Castor oil routines can be a small part of coping, but it should not replace deeper care if needed.

## 12. Safe Use Around Bedtime

When using castor oil at night, keep these points in mind:

- **Protect Bedding:** If you do a foot rub or a castor oil pack before bed, slip on old socks or place an old towel under you to avoid stains.
- **Watch for Slips:** If you get up at night, having oil on the soles of your feet might be slippery. Wearing socks or wiping your feet is wise.
- **Keep It Short:** A 15-30 minute routine can help. You do not need to spend hours.
- **Stay Warm:** If you feel chilly at night, adding a light blanket while you rest with a castor oil pack can be comforting.

## 13. Dealing with Racing Thoughts

Sometimes the mind will not switch off, even if you do something calming with castor oil. In that case, try pairing the castor oil step with a mental focus:

- **Count Your Breaths:** Breathe in for a count of four, hold for a second, and then out for a count of four.
- **Observe the Senses:** Notice the feeling of the oil on the skin, the warmth, or the slight pressure.
- **Repeat a Simple Phrase:** Something like "All is calm" in your head can help redirect anxious ideas.

These small mental tasks can keep your mind in the present moment, giving your thoughts less space to wander into worries.

---

## 14. Morning Stress vs. Evening Stress

Not all stress occurs at night. Some people wake up feeling tense because of the day's demands. If that is you, consider a quick castor oil foot rub in the morning. It might sound odd, but a short self-care act before starting the day could set a calmer tone. Or place a small warm pack on your upper back for 10 minutes to loosen tight muscles from sleep. The key is to adapt these ideas to the time of day you feel the most stress.

---

## 15. Combining Castor Oil with Other Relaxation Methods

1. **Warm Bath:** Soak for about 15 minutes, then do a castor oil foot rub.
2. **Gentle Stretches:** Loosen stiff muscles, then apply a small castor oil massage to the area.
3. **Low-Volume Music:** Some relaxing tunes can enhance the calm environment.
4. **Body Scan Exercise:** Mentally check each part of your body for tension while your feet soak in warm water mixed with a bit of castor oil.

When put together, these steps can create a calm atmosphere that helps you release stress slowly.

---

## 16. Handling Persistent Insomnia

If you have insomnia, meaning you regularly cannot sleep or stay asleep, castor oil might be one small part of the approach. However, chronic insomnia often has many causes: mental strain, poor sleep habits, or health conditions. A castor oil pack can help you relax, but you might also need to:

- Make your bedroom darker and quieter.
- Avoid caffeine late in the day.
- Limit screen time near bedtime.
- Speak with a sleep specialist if the problem continues.

There is no single fix for insomnia, but every gentle step can contribute to a better chance of rest.

---

## 17. Dealing with Restless Legs

Some folks experience a crawling or uncomfortable feeling in their legs at night, sometimes called restless leg syndrome. While castor oil has not been proven to fix this condition, a warm castor oil massage on the legs might reduce surface tension. If it helps you feel less restless, it may be worth trying. Still, consult a professional if restless legs disrupt your sleep often.

---

## 18. Castor Oil and Head-to-Toe Relaxation

One lesser-known trick is a slow "head-to-toe" approach with small amounts of castor oil:

1. **Forehead and Temples:** Lightly dab a drop of castor oil, rub in circles.
2. **Neck and Shoulders:** If you can reach, do gentle kneading.
3. **Arms and Hands:** Rub small circles on the wrists and palms.
4. **Abdomen:** Soft swirling motions, avoiding strong pressure.
5. **Legs and Feet:** End with slow foot rubs, as described earlier.

Each step can be brief, but the overall method might take about 10-15 minutes. By the end, you could feel a deeper sense of calm. Use small amounts of oil so you are not too greasy.

## 19. Could Castor Oil Packs Soothe Nighttime Tummy Upset?

Some people have mild digestive upset at night, which can keep them awake. A warm castor oil pack on the lower abdomen might ease mild tightness or spasms. It will not solve major issues, but for mild bloating or tension, the warmth could be relaxing. Pair that with sipping some warm water or an herbal tea (like chamomile) to calm the stomach. If nighttime digestive issues persist, consider checking your eating patterns or speaking with a healthcare provider.

---

## 20. Managing Stress from Work or School

In times of heavy mental work—like exam periods or project deadlines—your mind might spin with tasks. Carving out even 15 minutes at night to do a castor oil foot massage can be a small but meaningful act. It provides a boundary between your busy day and your rest time. You can say, "I will work until 9 PM, then I will shut off the computer, do a quick foot rub, and shift my mind toward relaxing." This boundary can help you recover enough to face the next day with a clearer head.

---

## 21. Watching Out for Allergic Reactions

Though castor oil is usually mild, stress can sometimes make your skin more sensitive. If you are trying castor oil for the first time, do a small patch test. Put a drop on your inner arm, wait a day, and see if there is any redness or itching. If you have no reaction, you can move on to bigger areas. If you notice irritation, discontinue use and consider another relaxation method.

## 22. Encouraging Family Relaxation

Some families use castor oil massages as a bonding activity—especially parents with children, using a gentle approach on the kids' feet or arms. This can be a calm end to a hectic day. But keep in mind:

- **Be Gentle:** Children's skin can be delicate, so use minimal pressure.
- **Use Tiny Amounts:** Children do not need much oil at all.
- **Check for Ticks and Rashes:** When rubbing the legs or feet, it is a chance to see if there are any bug bites, small scrapes, or dryness you missed before.
- **Safe Routine:** Do not let children handle the castor oil by themselves, as they might spill it or get it in their eyes.

This can create a calm setting before bedtime stories or lights out.

---

## 23. Planning for Travel or Busy Weeks

When traveling or facing a busy period, you might pack a small container of castor oil:

- **Foot Relief:** After walking all day, a quick rub can soothe tired feet.
- **Tense Neck:** If you have been sitting in a car or plane, a brief self-massage on the neck can help.
- **Quick Calm:** If a hotel room feels stressful, a warm washcloth with a few drops of castor oil on the abdomen might center you.

Being prepared in this way can keep stress from building to an uncomfortable level.

---

## 24. Real-Life Examples (No Names)

- **Case A:** A busy office worker realized that anxiety was affecting her sleep. She started rubbing castor oil on her feet each night while

practicing slow breathing. Within a week, she said she fell asleep faster and felt more rested.
- **Case B:** A college student used to watch videos until midnight, feeling restless. He swapped 15 minutes of screen time for a castor oil pack on his lower abdomen. He said the warm, quiet time helped him switch off, and he woke with more energy.

These are anecdotal stories, not clinical proof, but they hint at how simple changes can help.

---

## 25. Final Thoughts on Stress and Sleep Support

Stress and poor sleep can harm our well-being, so small steps that help calm the mind are valuable. Castor oil can be part of that. Whether you prefer a quick foot massage, a warm abdominal pack, or a gentle neck rub, the goal is to ease muscle tension and signal your brain that it is safe to slow down. Paired with mindful breathing, lower lights, and a phone-free bedtime, these acts can move you closer to restful sleep.

If stress or sleep issues are severe or last a long time, a simple oil routine may not be enough. In that case, it is wise to look for deeper help, such as professional counseling, therapy, or medical advice. But for many people, day-to-day tension can be reduced by creating short self-care moments. Castor oil is one tool that might help you find those moments of peace.

Now that we have looked at stress and sleep, our next chapters will go further into other ways that castor oil might assist with wellness, from easing muscles and joints to helping balance certain body functions. Yet always keep a broad approach to health: good nutrition, healthy movement, enough rest, and responsible advice from trusted professionals. By combining these, you can build a more balanced life, using simple items like castor oil as a friendly helper along the way.

# CHAPTER 11: JOINT AND MUSCLE RELIEF

Castor oil has a thick texture and a unique set of fats that may help support the body in different ways. One area where people often use it is for mild joint and muscle support. These are two places in the body that can become stressed from daily activities, aging, or physical strain. Some individuals say that rubbing castor oil on sore joints or stiff muscles helps them feel looser or more comfortable. In this chapter, we will explore why this might happen, how to apply castor oil for these purposes, and what safety points you need to keep in mind. While it is not a replacement for physical therapy or medical care, it might offer a simple, at-home measure for many people who want short-term comfort.

## 1. Basic View of Joints and Muscles

Joints are places where two bones meet. They allow us to bend, twist, and move in many ways. Between the bones is a space that normally holds fluid and cartilage, which help the bones move smoothly. Muscles pull on these bones to create motion, and they also help stabilize the joints. Over time, or after certain types of strain, these areas can hurt, swell, or feel stiff. Many factors may be involved: age, overuse, minor injury, or a health condition.

Muscles can become tight or overworked from exercise, repetitive motions, or sitting for long periods. Sometimes they ache from small tears that happen during workouts or from general tension. This tension can lead to a feeling of soreness that can make daily tasks harder.

## 2. Why People Think Castor Oil May Help

Castor oil has been used in folk remedies for quite some time to soothe mild joint or muscle aches. One reason might be that the thick oil helps keep warmth in when massaged onto the skin. Warmth often makes tight or stiff spots feel better. Another reason is ricinoleic acid, the main fatty acid in castor oil, which might help calm minor swelling in some people.

Researchers have looked at how ricinoleic acid interacts with tissues. Some lab studies suggest it can reduce certain signals that cause puffiness or redness in the body, though results can vary from person to person. Additionally, massaging the oil onto the skin can help improve blood flow locally, which may ease tension.

## 3. Common Ways to Use Castor Oil for Joint and Muscle Relief

1. **Direct Application:** The simplest method is rubbing a small amount of castor oil onto the target area. You can warm the oil slightly by placing the bottle in a bowl of warm water, then gently massaging it onto the skin.
2. **Castor Oil Packs:** These are pieces of cloth soaked in castor oil. You place the cloth over the joint or muscle, then cover it with plastic wrap or a towel. Adding gentle heat with a heating pad can make it feel even more soothing.
3. **Blended Massage Oils:** Some prefer to mix castor oil with lighter oils, such as almond or grapeseed, to make it easier to spread. This also helps avoid an overly heavy or sticky feel.
4. **Warm Baths with a Castor Oil Mix:** Though castor oil does not mix easily with water, some people like to combine it with a bit of Epsom salt or mild liquid soap. Then they add the mix to a warm bath, soaking the entire body. This might help with general muscle tightness.

## 4. Focus on Knees, Shoulders, and Hands

Certain joints, like knees, shoulders, and hands, are common trouble spots. Knees carry the weight of the body and bend often. Shoulders have a wide range of movement and can feel stiff if not stretched or if used too much.

Hands and fingers can become tight from typing or other repetitive tasks. Here is how castor oil might be used on each:

- **Knees:** Sit in a chair or lie down, then rub warm castor oil all around the knee. You can do gentle circles to massage the area. A castor oil pack might be placed on the knee for 15 to 30 minutes.
- **Shoulders:** If you can reach the spot, rub a small amount of oil around the shoulder socket. Some people find it easier to have someone help with the back of the shoulder. Light circular strokes may ease mild tightness.
- **Hands and Fingers:** Place a drop or two of castor oil in your palm, rub your hands together, and then focus on each finger joint. A gentle massage can help if you have minor stiffness from typing or manual work.

## 5. Adding Gentle Heat

Heat can improve how the oil feels and how it interacts with the skin. The warmth can also loosen tight muscles. You can use:

1. **A Heating Pad:** After applying castor oil, place a thin cloth over the area, then set a heating pad on low or medium. Check often to avoid burns.
2. **A Warm Towel:** Some people dip a towel in hot water, wring it out, and place it over the oiled joint or muscle. This can feel soothing, but you must be careful with the temperature.
3. **A Warm Bath or Shower First:** Taking a short warm bath or shower can open pores. Then, applying castor oil right after might help it soak in a bit better.

## 6. Joints vs. Muscles: Slight Differences in Approach

- **Joint Discomfort:** Often, individuals aim the oil at a specific area, like the knee or knuckles. They might use a pack to keep the oil and heat in place longer.

- **Muscle Soreness:** In contrast, muscle aches can cover a bigger area, such as the lower back or thighs. A gentle, slow massage with castor oil might be more practical. This helps spread the oil over a larger region.

Some people do both approaches if they have both joint and muscle complaints. For example, after a hard workout, someone's knees might be sore (joint focus), and their thighs might feel tight (muscle focus). They could use a castor oil pack on the knees, then do a broader oil massage on the thighs.

## 7. Working with Other Aids

Castor oil can be one of several ways to handle mild joint and muscle troubles. Others include:

1. **Stretching and Light Exercise:** Gentle movements can increase blood flow to stiff areas.
2. **Over-the-Counter Gels:** Some people use special rubs or gels with ingredients like menthol. You can alternate these with castor oil treatments if you find them helpful.
3. **Professional Massage:** Seeing a certified massage person can help with deeper tension. You could even ask them to use castor oil if they agree and if it suits their methods.
4. **Physical Therapy:** If the discomfort is more serious or related to an injury, physical therapy might be needed. Some PT sessions might allow you to use castor oil at home as part of your routine.

## 8. Tips for a Basic At-Home Castor Oil Massage

1. **Prepare the Area:** Clean the skin with mild soap and warm water. This removes dirt and helps the pores open.
2. **Warm the Oil:** As mentioned, place the bottle in a bowl of warm water for a few minutes.

3. **Apply a Small Amount:** Castor oil is thick, so a little goes a long way. You can always add more if needed.
4. **Use Gentle Pressure:** Firm, quick motions can cause discomfort. Slow, light-to-medium pressure helps soothe.
5. **Move in Circles:** This can help the oil spread evenly. Move outward from the center of pain if it is a muscle area, or around the joint in small loops if it is a joint.
6. **Consider a Short Break Afterward:** Sit or lie down quietly for a few minutes to let the area rest. Cover it with a towel if you do not want the oil getting on clothes.

---

## 9. Frequency of Use

How often can you use castor oil for joints or muscles? It varies:

- **Mild Soreness:** Once or twice a week might be enough.
- **More Regular Stiffness:** Some people do a short application daily or every other day.
- **Post-Workout:** If you are very active, applying castor oil after high-intensity sessions may help you relax.

Listen to your body. If daily use seems too much, cut back. If once a week helps but does not keep soreness away, you might try twice a week. Avoid over-reliance on any single remedy if you are not seeing improvement over time.

---

## 10. Precautions and Warnings

1. **Serious Joint Problems:** If you have significant swelling, redness, or extreme pain, see a professional. Castor oil cannot replace medical tests or targeted treatments.
2. **Broken Skin:** If you have cuts or open sores near a painful joint or muscle, do not apply castor oil without checking with a health worker. The oil might trap bacteria or cause irritation.
3. **Allergies:** Rare, but possible. If you notice rashes or itchiness, stop using castor oil.

4. **Heat Sensitivity:** Some older adults or those with nerve issues might not feel heat properly. They should be careful with heating pads so they do not burn themselves.

## 11. Combining with Gentle Movement Routines

Basic movement can help loosen muscles and keep joints limber. Some people do small exercises right after applying castor oil (or after a castor oil pack session), believing that the warmth from the oil and the increased circulation make gentle stretching easier. Here are some ideas:

- **Neck Rolls:** If you have tight neck muscles, applying castor oil, then lightly rolling the neck from side to side might help.
- **Shoulder Rolls:** After rubbing castor oil on the shoulders, do slow forward and backward shoulder rolls.
- **Knee Bends:** If your knees feel stiff, carefully try mini squats or just a few slow bends (without overdoing it).
- **Wrist Circles:** For the hands, rub the oil in, then do gentle wrist circles and finger stretches.

Never force a motion if it hurts, and consult a professional if you have a specific injury.

## 12. Could Castor Oil Help with Tension in the Back?

The back is a mix of many muscles and joints along the spine. While castor oil might not fix underlying disc or nerve problems, it could help soothe mild tightness in the back muscles:

1. **Lower Back Packs:** People who sit a lot might place a castor oil pack on the lower back for 20-30 minutes. They could add gentle heat to relax stiff tissue.
2. **Shoulder Blade Massage:** If you can reach between the shoulder blades, you can do a light rub there, or ask someone to help you.
3. **Wide Coverage:** Because the back is large, you may need to blend castor oil with another oil to spread it more easily.

If back pain is constant or severe, check with a health professional. Sometimes it might be related to posture, a pinched nerve, or another issue that needs specialized attention.

---

## 13. Helping the Body's Self-Healing

When we use mild approaches like castor oil, we are often supporting the body's own ability to relax and recover from daily strain. By adding warmth, improving local blood flow, and reducing mild swelling, we can assist the natural healing process. The body repairs small muscle tears and tries to keep joints lubricated. These small steps might help you avoid heavier treatments for everyday aches.

This does not mean castor oil is a miracle. It is one piece in a larger puzzle of good health habits: balanced food, enough rest, suitable movement, and sometimes professional therapies. The goal is to keep small problems from becoming big ones.

---

## 14. Simple Recipes for Joint and Muscle Salves

You can make a homemade salve that includes castor oil. Here is a basic idea:

- **Ingredients:** 2 tablespoons of castor oil, 2 tablespoons of another carrier oil (like coconut), 1 tablespoon of beeswax (to create a balm texture).
- **Steps:**
    1. Melt beeswax in a double boiler on low heat.
    2. Stir in castor oil and the other carrier oil until well combined.
    3. Pour into a small container and let it cool.

Once it sets, you have a balm. You can rub it on knees, elbows, or any muscle area that feels tight. Some people add a drop of mild essential oil, like peppermint (for a cooling feel) or lavender (for a gentle scent), but that is optional. Always do a patch test if you add essential oils.

## 15. How to Tell If It's Working

If you apply castor oil to a stiff muscle or joint, how do you know it is helping?

- **Short-Term Relief:** You might feel less tightness or a soothing warmth in the area.
- **Improved Movement:** If a knee was stiff, you might notice slightly easier bending after you finish.
- **Less Tension:** The area may not ache as much when you do daily tasks.

This relief might be subtle or might only last for a few hours. Continued gentle use, plus other supportive steps (like mild exercise), might extend these benefits. If the tightness is linked to a deeper issue, you might need more specialized care.

## 16. Doing a Full Leg Massage

For people who have soreness from running or other sports, a full leg massage can help:

1. **Gather Supplies:** You will need a towel, warmed castor oil (maybe mixed with a lighter oil), and something to sit on comfortably.
2. **Start at the Ankles:** Use upward strokes to move blood flow toward the heart.
3. **Focus on Calves:** Use both hands in a gentle, kneading motion. Calves can become tight, especially if you have been walking or running a lot.
4. **Move to the Thighs:** Continue the upward strokes, taking care around sensitive areas.
5. **Finish at the Hips:** If you can, massage around the hip area lightly. Avoid pressing on the hip bones too firmly.
6. **Pat Off Excess Oil:** When done, lightly dab with a towel. Put on loose clothing to let the skin breathe.

## 17. Evening Routine for Muscle Recovery

If you have minor muscle aches from a day of chores, work, or light exercise, you might try:

- **Warm Shower:** This helps relax the muscles and open pores.
- **Castor Oil Massage:** Focus on the main areas that feel strained—maybe shoulders, arms, or legs.
- **Stretch or Do Easy Yoga Moves:** Just a few slow poses to keep the muscles from tightening again.
- **Rest with a Warm Cloth:** You could place a warm, damp towel over the area for 10 minutes.

Then go about your night routine. This can help you wake up with fewer aches the next morning.

## 18. Balancing Activity and Rest

While castor oil might soothe joints and muscles, remember the importance of balancing movement with rest. Overworking a joint or muscle can lead to more pain. Underusing them can also cause stiffness. A moderate routine that includes regular walking, gentle stretching, and breaks from prolonged sitting can prevent some of the soreness that leads you to reach for castor oil in the first place.

## 19. Using Castor Oil After Minor Injuries

If you twist an ankle or strain a muscle, the usual advice is to rest, ice, compress, and elevate (R.I.C.E) in the first day or two. Once swelling goes down, some people add a warm castor oil rub for mild comfort. But you have to be sure the main swelling phase has passed. Putting heat on a fresh injury can worsen swelling. Always follow guidelines for the specific type of injury, and if in doubt, ask a health worker.

## 20. Myths vs. Reality

1. **"Castor Oil Heals All Joint Diseases"**: Not true. It might help minor aches, but joint diseases often need professional management.
2. **"More Oil Means Faster Relief"**: You do not need to soak yourself in castor oil. A thin layer is usually enough.
3. **"All Pain Disappears Instantly"**: Some relief might be quick, but deep issues need more thorough solutions.

Staying grounded in what castor oil can and cannot do will help you get the most out of it without expecting miracles.

---

## 21. Observing Changes Over Time

If you plan to use castor oil packs or massages regularly for a few weeks, consider noting how you feel:

- **Intensity of Discomfort:** Is it mild, moderate, or severe each day?
- **Range of Motion:** Can you bend or move more smoothly than before?
- **Daily Activities:** Are tasks like climbing stairs or opening jars easier after consistent use?

This informal tracking can help you decide whether castor oil is worth including in your long-term approach or if you should try something else.

---

## 22. Speaking with Health Professionals

If you have a long-standing muscle or joint issue, do not rely solely on home remedies. A doctor or physical therapist can check if there is an underlying problem, like cartilage wear or muscle imbalances. They may suggest specific exercises, braces, or even certain nutritional strategies. You can mention that you are trying castor oil. They might have thoughts about how to fit it into a broader care plan.

## 23. Helping Stiff Neck Muscles at the Desk

Many people spend hours on the computer or phone, leading to a stiff neck and tight upper back. A small bottle of castor oil at your desk might be handy, but be careful not to get oil on your clothes. You can do a quick rub on your neck and shoulders during a break:

1. **Stand Up and Roll Shoulders:** Loosen up first.
2. **Apply a Drop of Castor Oil on Fingertips:** Massage your neck gently, focusing on tight spots.
3. **Stretch:** Tilt your head side to side slowly.
4. **Wipe Off Any Excess Oil:** Use a tissue or cloth.

Even a few minutes can help break up tension.

## 24. Considerations for Sports Enthusiasts

If you are involved in sports like soccer, basketball, or running, minor muscle aches are part of the routine. A castor oil rub might be something you add to your cooldown process. However, keep in mind:

- **Sweaty Skin:** Wash off sweat first. Castor oil on dirty or sweaty skin can trap dirt.
- **Allow Time to Absorb:** If you need to put on compression wear afterward, the oil might stain.
- **Not a Substitute for Stretching and Hydration:** Proper cooldown, water intake, and muscle-friendly meals are still the main supports.

# CHAPTER 12: HORMONE BALANCE

Castor oil is often associated with external applications, such as skin care or muscle relief. However, some people also talk about a possible link between castor oil and hormone balance. Hormones are chemical messengers that influence many functions in the body, including growth, mood, reproduction, and energy levels. When hormones become imbalanced, it can lead to issues like mood swings, changes in menstrual cycles, or other challenges. In this chapter, we will explore how some individuals use castor oil packs or other methods to help support normal hormone functions. We will review traditional ideas, theories about how castor oil might affect the body, and the limits of what we currently know. As always, for serious hormone concerns, you should seek professional guidance.

## 1. What Are Hormones?

Hormones are substances that glands in the body release into the bloodstream. These glands include the thyroid, adrenal glands, ovaries, testes, and others. The hormones they produce can affect how cells behave. Examples include:

- **Estrogen and Progesterone:** Important for women's reproductive cycles and other roles.
- **Testosterone:** Linked with muscle mass, libido, and other functions.
- **Thyroid Hormones:** Affect metabolism and energy use.
- **Cortisol:** Related to stress responses.
- **Insulin:** Controls blood sugar levels.

A steady balance of these hormones helps the body work smoothly. When there are major shifts or imbalances, a person might notice things like irregular cycles, tiredness, mood changes, or weight shifts. Many factors can influence hormone levels, such as diet, stress, age, and certain health conditions.

## 2. Why People Connect Castor Oil to Hormone Balance

Some alternative health views suggest that castor oil packs placed on certain areas of the abdomen (like over the reproductive organs or the liver) may help the body handle hormones better. One idea is that castor oil packs might encourage healthy blood flow and lymph flow, allowing the body to process hormones or remove excess hormones more effectively. Another line of thought is that castor oil might soothe mild swelling in the area, helping tissues function at their best.

There is also talk about how the liver, which helps break down hormones once they have served their purpose, might get a mild boost when a person uses warm castor oil packs on the right side of the abdomen. As mentioned in Chapter 9, though, we do not have large-scale research proving that castor oil directly balances hormones. Most of these ideas come from personal experiences or small groups that share tips.

## 3. Possible Areas to Place Castor Oil Packs for Hormone Support

1. **Lower Abdomen:** Some place a castor oil pack here to cover the uterus and ovaries (for women) or just the lower digestive region. They believe it could help with menstrual comfort or minor bloating.
2. **Liver Area (Right Side):** Because the liver processes hormones, some people put a castor oil pack on the right upper abdomen, hoping to support the breakdown and clearance of old hormones.
3. **Lower Back (Near Kidneys):** Others think that overall fluid balance and stress reduction might help hormone health. They might place a pack here for comfort.

Again, these methods are more based on tradition and personal stories rather than confirmed findings. If you choose to do this, see it as a gentle practice, not a guaranteed fix.

## 4. Menstrual Support

Some women use castor oil packs to help with mild menstrual discomfort or irregular cycles. A common approach is:

1. **Days Before the Cycle:** They apply a warm castor oil pack on the lower abdomen for 20-30 minutes each day, except during menstruation if the flow is heavy.
2. **Mild Heat:** The warmth might reduce muscle tightness.
3. **Relaxation:** The quiet time can lower stress, which sometimes plays a role in hormone fluctuations.

If you have severe menstrual pain, unusual bleeding, or suspect other issues, it is wise to see a healthcare worker. Castor oil may help mild cramps but is not a solution for major problems.

---

## 5. Polycystic Ovary Syndrome (PCOS) and Related Issues

PCOS is a condition that can affect hormone levels, leading to irregular cycles, unwanted hair growth, and sometimes difficulties with fertility. There is no proof that castor oil cures PCOS. Some users, though, say a warm pack on the lower abdomen offers mild comfort or relaxation. If you have PCOS, your treatment might include lifestyle changes, certain medicines, or other measures. Castor oil packs could be a small add-on if they help you relax.

---

## 6. Thyroid Concerns

The thyroid gland is in the neck and controls metabolism. When it is underactive or overactive, problems can arise. Some people wonder if applying castor oil packs to the neck area might help. However, the neck is a delicate region. Using thick oil and heat there needs extra care. We do not have strong evidence that castor oil can change thyroid hormone production. If you suspect a thyroid imbalance (like fatigue, weight changes, or temperature sensitivity), get tested by a medical professional.

## 7. Stress and Hormones

Stress can throw off hormone levels, including cortisol and sometimes sex hormones. A big part of stress management involves good sleep, balanced activity, and a calm mind. We discussed in Chapter 10 how castor oil packs and massages might help a person relax. This relaxation could indirectly help the body's stress hormones settle. By calming tension, you might see mild improvements in how your body feels overall. But castor oil alone cannot fix deep stress problems or serious hormone shifts from chronic stress. Think of it as part of a set of calming steps.

## 8. Possible Role of Lymphatic Movement

The lymphatic system carries waste and helps the immune system. Some believe that if the lymph flow is slow, the body may have trouble removing extra hormones or byproducts. Castor oil packs might support local lymph flow by warming the area and increasing circulation. However, this idea is mostly based on personal accounts. If you think sluggish lymph is part of your hormone concerns, ask a health worker how to handle it. Exercise, staying hydrated, and occasional gentle massage can also help keep lymph fluid moving.

## 9. Balancing Hormones Naturally: A Wider Perspective

If you are looking to help hormone balance, remember that castor oil is just one tiny piece. Other helpful steps include:

1. **Proper Nutrition:** Eating balanced meals with proteins, healthy fats, and a variety of fruits and vegetables can support hormone production and breakdown.

2. **Regular Movement:** Exercise helps your body regulate hormones like insulin and can lower stress hormones.
3. **Adequate Sleep:** Many hormones, including those linked to growth and repair, are influenced by how well you rest.
4. **Limiting Harmful Substances:** Too much alcohol or a very high-sugar diet can strain your system.
5. **Checking Medications and Supplements:** Some pills or supplements can affect hormone levels.

Castor oil might be a gentle support, but the main actions usually happen through daily habits.

---

## 10. Castor Oil and Fertility

Some people wonder if castor oil packs can help with fertility. The idea is that improving blood flow around the reproductive organs might help create a more welcoming environment. However, there is no conclusive research proving this. Fertility can be complex, involving many factors, such as age, overall health, timing, and possible medical conditions. If you and a partner are trying to conceive and facing challenges, talk to a qualified doctor. Castor oil packs could be an optional relaxation technique, but relying on them alone may not be enough.

---

## 11. Safe Use of Castor Oil for Hormone Support

- **Avoid Internal Use for This Purpose:** Drinking castor oil can cause strong bowel movements and is not recommended as a hormone-balancing method.
- **Use Packs or Rubs Externally:** Keep the oil on your skin over the area you want to support.
- **Short Sessions:** Most users do 20-30 minutes. Some might go up to an hour. Overdoing it is not likely to speed results and may irritate the skin.

- **Follow Your Cycle:** If you are a woman who wants to use castor oil packs for menstrual comfort, track your cycle and see which days it feels most helpful.

## 12. Signs Your Hormones Might Be Off

While only lab tests can confirm hormone levels, some signs that you might want to check with a professional include:

- **Sudden Weight Changes:** Gaining or losing without a clear reason.
- **Extreme Fatigue:** Feeling exhausted even when you have slept enough.
- **Mood Swings or Anxiety:** Especially if they do not match your usual patterns.
- **Irregular Periods or Absent Periods:** For women of reproductive age.
- **Hair Loss or Excess Hair Growth:** If it happens quickly or in an unusual pattern.
- **Skin Changes:** Sudden acne or dryness that does not improve.

Castor oil packs might soothe some mild aches or tension, but they cannot diagnose or correct major hormone imbalances on their own.

## 13. Making Castor Oil Pack Routines for Hormone Health

If you decide to try castor oil packs for hormone-related reasons, you might create a schedule. For instance:

1. **Once or Twice a Week:** Choose a time in the evening when you can lie down for 30 minutes uninterrupted.
2. **Focus on the Lower Abdomen or the Right Side:** Depending on whether you want to support the reproductive organs or the liver.
3. **Gentle Heat:** Put a heating pad or warm towel on top.
4. **Quiet Activity:** Read a calming book or listen to light music.

5. **Stay Hydrated:** Drink water or herbal tea afterward.

Keep track of how you feel over a month or two, but remember that hormone shifts can take time. If you see no change, or if things get worse, consider speaking with a professional.

---

## 14. Mixing Castor Oil with Mild Herbs

Some alternative approaches include adding mild herbs to a castor oil pack. For example, someone might soak the cloth in castor oil and add a few drops of herb-infused oil like chamomile or rosemary. The idea is that the blend can add extra calming or supportive properties. However, there is limited data on how these mixes affect hormones. Also, be cautious with essential oils if you have sensitive skin. Always test a small area first.

---

## 15. Stress Hormones and Castor Oil

Cortisol is a main stress hormone. If you are constantly stressed, cortisol levels can remain high or become imbalanced, leading to issues like disturbed sleep or changes in appetite. Using castor oil packs for relaxation, as noted in previous chapters, might help you find a calmer state before bed or after a hectic day. Over time, lowering stress might help your body handle cortisol better. This is not a direct chemical action of castor oil on cortisol, but rather a result of giving yourself a break and letting the body calm down.

---

## 16. Supports for Men's Hormones

Men also have hormone fluctuations, though not as cyclical as women's. Testosterone levels can dip due to stress, poor sleep, or other factors. While castor oil packs are talked about more in the context of women's health, men might also use them for abdominal relaxation, especially if they face mild digestive stress or tension that could indirectly affect hormones.

However, we do not have specific proof that castor oil directly raises or stabilizes testosterone.

---

## 17. Safe Use for Pregnant or Breastfeeding Women?

Hormone changes during pregnancy and postpartum are significant. Some mothers wonder if castor oil packs can help them bounce back or maintain balance. However, most sources say to be careful with castor oil during pregnancy because swallowing it can stimulate strong bowel contractions or even uterine contractions. For external packs, it might be less risky, but it is still wise to talk to a healthcare worker. During breastfeeding, applying castor oil on the abdomen might not be harmful, but again, check with a doctor to be sure.

---

## 18. Castor Oil Packs vs. Professional Hormone Treatments

If you have a confirmed hormone issue, like hypothyroidism, insulin resistance, or severe estrogen imbalance, a doctor might give you medications (like thyroid hormone replacement or birth control pills) or specific therapies. Castor oil packs are not a substitute for these treatments. They might make you feel more comfortable or relaxed, but they do not replace blood tests, prescribed hormone pills, or ongoing medical supervision.

---

## 19. Emotional Well-Being and Hormones

Hormone issues can affect mood. Some people notice that when they do regular castor oil pack sessions, they feel calmer emotionally. This may be from the pause in a busy schedule, the mild warmth, or the sense of caring for oneself. Emotional well-being is tied to hormones like serotonin and cortisol, so any calming routine can help in an indirect way. However, if you have serious mood swings or signs of depression, professional help is key.

## 20. Myths About Castor Oil Curing All Hormone Woes

1. **"It Immediately Balances Hormones"**: The body's hormone system is complex. Castor oil cannot instantly fix imbalances.
2. **"You Don't Need Lifestyle Changes"**: Some claim that castor oil alone can solve hormone problems, but ignore diet, stress, or medical conditions. That is not realistic.
3. **"All Women Must Use Castor Oil for Menstrual Health"**: Some women never use it and have normal cycles. Others try it and see mild benefits. It is a personal choice, not a must-do for everyone.

## 21. Observing Subtle Shifts

If you are using castor oil packs to support normal hormone function, be patient. Hormones can shift over weeks or months. You might keep a journal of your daily energy, mood, or cycle patterns. Note when you use the castor oil pack, how long, and where. Over time, see if there is any pattern. If you feel a bit more stable or your cycle is less uncomfortable, it might be one sign that your overall approach (including the pack) is helping. If you notice no change at all, or negative changes, you might stop the method or talk to a professional.

## 22. Time of Day for Hormone-Related Packs

Some people believe that doing castor oil packs in the evening helps them rest, which indirectly supports hormone regulation overnight. Others do them in the morning, saying they feel more balanced for the day. There is no strict rule. You can pick a time that fits your schedule. Just make sure you can sit or lie quietly for the session. If you have daily chores or kids running around, you might prefer a time when interruptions are minimal.

## 23. Combining Packs with Light Abdominal Massage

If you want to focus on the lower abdomen (for menstrual or general hormone support):

1. **Warm the Oil:** Soak your cloth in warmed castor oil.
2. **Place Over Lower Belly:** Gently lay it from below the navel to the pubic area.
3. **Add Heat (Optional):** Put a heating pad on low.
4. **Abdominal Massage:** After 10-15 minutes, you can remove the pack briefly to do a slow, clockwise massage around the belly button. Some believe this helps with bowel movements and lightens tension. Then you can reapply the pack if you wish.

---

## 24. Alternative Approaches

Other non-castor oil ways to support hormone balance could include:

- **Herbal Teas:** Some claim herbs like raspberry leaf or chasteberry might support hormone rhythms, though evidence varies.
- **Mind-Body Practices:** Yoga, easy meditation, or slow breathing can calm stress responses that affect hormones.
- **Supplements:** Sometimes vitamins or minerals (like vitamin D or magnesium) can help if you are low. Get tested or ask a professional.
- **Counseling for Stress:** Chronic stress can harm hormone health, so working on the mental side can be vital.

If you mix these methods with castor oil packs, make sure you do not overload yourself. Start slowly, track any changes, and keep an eye on how you feel.

# CHAPTER 13: HOME REMEDIES FOR PARENTS AND CHILDREN

Castor oil has long been part of family traditions in certain households. From mild skin care to small comfort measures, parents sometimes search for natural options that can be used safely with children. While caution is always needed with any product, castor oil can be handy for a variety of small home remedies. In this chapter, we will look at ways parents might use castor oil for themselves and their kids, how to do it safely, and when it is best to seek professional help. We will also talk about specific points, like dosages or external applications, and tips on introducing castor oil in a child-friendly manner.

## 1. Safety First: General Guidelines

Before looking at specific uses, we need to remember that children's bodies are more sensitive than adults'. What might be fine for a grown-up can be too strong for a small child. Here are some key reminders:

1. **Patch Test:** If you plan to use castor oil on a child's skin, test a tiny drop on the inside of the child's forearm. Wait 24 hours to see if there is any redness or itching. If there is none, it is likely safe to use in a larger area.
2. **No Raw Seeds:** Never let a child handle raw castor seeds. They contain harmful substances. Only use professionally made castor oil, which has had toxins removed or deactivated.
3. **Avoid Oral Use for Young Children:** It is generally not advised to give small children castor oil to swallow for constipation or other internal uses, unless a health worker says otherwise. Children can become dehydrated more easily if they have diarrhea or strong bowel movements.

4. **Observe and Monitor:** Even with safe external use, watch the child for any changes. Kids might not always say if something feels itchy or hot. Look at the skin for signs of redness.
5. **Small Amounts:** A little castor oil is enough in most cases. Using large amounts may cause mess, staining, or discomfort.

---

## 2. Soothing Dry Skin in Children

Children can get dry patches on their skin, such as on the cheeks, elbows, or knees. Some might have mild forms of sensitive or easily irritated skin. Castor oil's thickness can create a protective layer:

1. **Application Method:**
   - Wash and dry the child's skin gently with mild soap and water.
   - Put a small drop of castor oil on your fingertip.
   - Rub it in a slow, circular motion onto the dry patch.
   - If it still feels too oily after a few minutes, pat off the excess with a clean cloth.
2. **Frequency:** You might do this once a day if needed, perhaps after a bath. That way, the skin can hold onto moisture better. If the dry patch improves, you can reduce the frequency.
3. **Caution:** If the dry patch is cracked or if there is any sign of infection (like redness, swelling, or fluid), seek advice rather than trying to solve it at home. Castor oil can help dryness, but open or infected skin may need professional care.

---

## 3. Mild Support for Itchy Bug Bites

Kids are often active and can get bug bites. Some parents apply a little castor oil to a bite, hoping it will reduce the itch:

1. **Clean the Bite Area:** Gently wash with mild soap and water.
2. **Dab on the Oil:** Use a cotton swab to place a tiny spot of castor oil directly on the bite.

3. **Observe:** Watch for any change. If the child feels relief, great. If it gets more red or the child complains of increasing discomfort, stop using it and consider another approach.

Sometimes castor oil's thickness can keep the area from drying out, which might reduce minor irritation. But for serious reactions or large swelling, talk to a professional.

---

## 4. Castor Oil Foot Rub for Calming

Many children have busy days filled with school, sports, or playtime. Some parents find that a short foot rub before bedtime can help a child wind down:

1. **Setting the Scene:**
    - Have the child wash their feet in warm water.
    - Dry them well.
    - Sit together in a calm space, maybe the living room or the child's bedroom.
2. **How to Massage:**
    - Put a pea-sized drop of castor oil in your palm.
    - Gently rub the bottoms of the child's feet, focusing on the arch and heel.
    - Use slow, circular motions. Keep the pressure gentle.
3. **Optional Socks:** If you do this near bedtime, you can have the child wear cotton socks afterward to keep the sheets clean. Some kids enjoy the cozy feel, while others prefer bare feet.
4. **Keep It Short and Comfortable:** About one or two minutes per foot can be enough. The main purpose is a small moment of calm. This routine can also be a bonding activity.

---

## 5. Tummy Comfort: Warm Castor Oil Pack

Older children might complain of mild tummy aches from time to time, often linked to gas or general discomfort. Some parents consider a gentle castor oil pack for the abdomen. However, be sure the child is not dealing with a more serious issue like appendicitis or food poisoning. For mild, normal tummy complaints:

1. **Prepare a Warm Pack:**
   - Warm a small amount of castor oil in a bowl of warm water (do not make it hot).
   - Take a soft cloth and soak it in the oil.
   - Squeeze out any extra to avoid dripping.
2. **Apply on the Abdomen:**
   - Have the child lie down on their back.
   - Place the cloth on the lower or middle belly, wherever they feel discomfort.
   - Cover the cloth with plastic wrap or a dry towel to prevent mess.
3. **Add Mild Heat (Optional):**
   - You can place a warm (not hot) water bottle on top for 10-15 minutes. Watch closely so it does not get too warm for the child.
4. **Check for Improvement:** If the child feels better, great. If pain persists or worsens, remove the pack and consider another approach or seek professional guidance.

---

# 6. Gentle Help with Hair Tangles

Kids with curly or long hair often struggle with tangles. A few drops of castor oil, blended with a lighter oil or a hair conditioner, can help loosen knots:

1. **Mixing:** In a small bowl, combine one teaspoon of castor oil with one tablespoon of a lighter oil (such as coconut or olive) or a mild conditioner.
2. **Dab on Tangles:** While the child's hair is damp (after a bath), apply the mixture to the ends or the knotted areas.
3. **Comb Slowly:** Use a wide-tooth comb. Start at the ends, working upward. The oil mixture can help the comb glide.

Be careful not to apply too much near the scalp, as it can leave the hair looking heavy or oily. Also, avoid contact with the child's eyes.

## 7. Mild Support for Nasal Dryness (External Use Only)

Some kids get dry skin around the nostrils in colder weather or if they blow their nose often. You can dab a very small amount of castor oil around the outside of the nostril openings to soften dry skin. Do not put castor oil inside the nasal passages unless a health professional advises it. Keep it strictly external. This can help reduce cracked or sore spots that come from frequent wiping.

## 8. Lip Care for Children

Children's lips can become chapped from playing outside, especially in windy or cold conditions. A tiny bit of castor oil on the lips can form a protective layer. If the child licks their lips a lot, though, it is better to use a mild lip balm that tastes more pleasant. Castor oil can have a strong taste. Still, if you only have castor oil on hand:

1. **Clean Lips:** Gently wipe them with a soft cloth.
2. **Apply a Very Thin Layer:** Use your fingertip or a cotton swab to spread a small amount of castor oil.
3. **Remind Child Not to Lick:** The flavor might be off-putting, and frequent licking can worsen dryness.

## 9. Short Massage for Growing Pains

Children sometimes experience "growing pains" in the legs at night, often in the calves or thighs. While these pains are not fully understood, many parents find that massaging the area can help calm the child:

1. **Rub Warm Castor Oil:**

- Warm a tablespoon of castor oil by placing the bottle or a small bowl in warm water.
- Gently massage the thighs or calves where the child says it aches.
2. **Short Session:** 2-3 minutes of slow rubbing might be enough.
3. **Comfort and Reassurance:** Growing pains can be upsetting. Quiet words and a gentle hug can help the child relax.

Of course, if pains are severe or frequent, check with a medical worker to rule out other causes.

## 10. Mild Constipation in Older Kids (With Caution)

As mentioned earlier, giving castor oil by mouth to children can be strong. It is safer to try other methods for mild constipation in kids. However, in some cases, a health professional might approve a tiny dose for an older child. If that happens:

1. **Exact Dose:** Follow the professional's directions carefully. Do not guess.
2. **Mix with Juice:** If the taste is too strong, a small amount can be mixed into a sweet juice.
3. **Stay Hydrated:** Keep the child drinking water to prevent dehydration.
4. **Watch for Cramping:** If the child complains of pain, speak to the professional again.

It is crucial not to use castor oil too often or in large amounts. If a child regularly struggles with constipation, a doctor or dietitian might suggest increasing fiber or using gentler options.

## 11. Using Castor Oil in Homemade Balms for Children

Some parents like to make simple balms to keep on hand for small scrapes or rough skin patches. Castor oil can be added to these mixes:

1. **Basic Recipe:**
   - 1 tablespoon beeswax pellets
   - 1 tablespoon castor oil
   - 1 tablespoon coconut oil or olive oil
2. **Steps:**
   - Melt the beeswax in a double boiler on low heat.
   - Stir in castor oil and the other oil until everything is combined.
   - Remove from heat and pour into small, clean containers.
   - Let it cool. The balm will solidify.
3. **Application:** Use a small dab on dry knuckles or mild skin spots. This is for external use only, so do not use it on open wounds or near the eyes.

Label the balm container and store it in a cool, dry place. It can be a convenient item in your family's kit.

---

## 12. Care Around the Eyes

Children might rub their eyes frequently, especially if they are tired or if something is bothering them. A small number of adults use castor oil on eyelashes or eyelids, but with kids, caution is extra important. If you consider using castor oil near the eyes for dryness on the eyelids (externally only):

1. **Tiny Amount:** Only use a fraction of a drop, and keep it on the eyelid skin, away from the eye.
2. **Explain to the Child:** Let them know not to rub their eyes afterward.
3. **Watch Closely:** If any oil gets in the eye, rinse with clean water. Though castor oil is not as harsh as some chemicals, it can still blur vision and may irritate sensitive eyes.

# 13. Helping Parents, Too

Parents often get tired or stressed. Castor oil can help them as well:

- **Foot Rub After a Long Day:** A quick self-massage or having a partner massage your feet with castor oil can be relaxing.
- **Hand Care:** Washing dishes or cleaning the house can dry out hands. Rubbing a drop of castor oil can soothe dryness. Put on light gloves for a short while if you do not want to get oil on surfaces.
- **Mild Neck Tension:** For tension at the base of the neck, rub in circles with a small amount of warm castor oil. Wipe off extra so you do not stain clothes.

When parents feel more at ease, they are better able to handle the demands of caring for children. Simple steps can make a difference in day-to-day well-being.

---

# 14. Bonding Through Mini Self-Care Sessions

Some families schedule short "mini spa" times. They might do face rinses, quick foot soaks, or gentle hand massages. Castor oil can be part of these sessions:

1. **Hand Soak:**
   - Fill a small bowl with warm water.
   - Add a drop of mild soap.
   - Have everyone soak their hands for a minute or two.
   - Dry them, then rub castor oil on the backs of the hands to seal in moisture.
2. **Foot Soak:**
   - A small tub of warm water for each child (or share one if it is large enough).
   - After drying, apply a pea-sized drop of castor oil to each foot.
   - You can chat or tell short stories while doing this.

These simple acts can bring a sense of togetherness and teach children about gentle self-care without needing expensive products.

## 15. Storing Castor Oil at Home

Be sure to keep your castor oil bottle in a safe place, out of children's reach. They might be curious about it. Store it in a cool, dark cabinet. Check that the cap is sealed to prevent leaks or accidents. If you have a child who likes to explore, consider placing it on a higher shelf. Always supervise young kids if you are using the oil around them.

## 16. Communicating with Older Children

Older children or teens might be curious about how to use castor oil for their own hair or skin. If so, explain the following:

- **Less Is More:** Castor oil is thick, so start with small amounts.
- **Never Drink It Without Guidance:** Oral use can be harsh. They should not try it as a "cleanse" they see online.
- **Be Consistent, Not Excessive:** If they want to use it for hair ends or dry elbows, a short routine once or twice a week is usually enough.

Helping them learn how to care for themselves responsibly can foster healthy habits later on.

## 17. Recognizing When to Seek Help

Castor oil is not a cure for serious health problems. As a parent, you need to watch for signs that a child might have a condition beyond a simple home remedy:

- **High Fever:** If the child has a fever that will not go down, do not rely on castor oil packs. See a health worker.

- **Persistent Pain or Swelling:** Ongoing pain in the belly, joints, or anywhere else needs professional review.
- **Allergic Reactions:** If you see hives, severe itchiness, or swelling, stop using castor oil immediately and get medical advice.
- **Long-Term Skin Issues:** If dryness or rashes last for weeks, there might be an underlying cause. A doctor's input is best.

Knowing the limits of home care helps keep children safe and ensures they receive proper treatment when needed.

---

## 18. Quick Remedies for Everyday Mishaps

Families deal with small issues daily—like a minor bump, slight bruise, or mild muscle soreness after sports. While castor oil cannot fix a bruise instantly, some parents like to rub a drop around (not on broken skin) to keep the area from drying out:

1. **For Bruises:**
    - Gently wash the area.
    - If it is fresh, some prefer a cool compress.
    - Later, if the skin is intact, a small castor oil rub might help keep the skin soft.
2. **For Mild Muscle Twinges:**
    - A short rub can help comfort the child.
    - Encourage light stretching or rest if the muscle is sore from overuse.
3. **Headaches (Older Children):**
    - Very gentle massage at the temples with a tiny dab of castor oil can be calming, though not all kids like the smell or sensation.

---

## 19. Fun Crafts or Projects

Sometimes kids might see an adult using castor oil and ask what it is for. A fun project is creating a simple lip balm or lotion bar together, as long as you supervise the heating steps:

1. **Lip Balm Bar:**
   - Melt 1 tablespoon beeswax, 1 teaspoon castor oil, and 1 teaspoon coconut oil.
   - Add a drop of vanilla extract (food-grade) if desired for scent.
   - Pour into small lip balm containers. Let it cool.
   - Label it, so the child knows it is for lips only.
2. **Hand Lotion Bar:**
   - Melt 2 tablespoons beeswax, 1 tablespoon castor oil, and 1 tablespoon shea butter.
   - Pour into a mold (like a silicone muffin cup).
   - Once it cools, you have a solid bar to rub on dry hands.

Kids often enjoy seeing how these items are made and using something they helped create.

## 20. Navigating Peer Advice and Online Tips

Older kids, especially teens, might read about castor oil "cures" online. As a parent, it helps to have open conversations about what they find:

- **Check the Source:** Remind them that not all online tips come from reliable places.
- **Balance and Moderation:** Even natural products can be harmful if misused.
- **Ask for Help:** Encourage them to talk to you or another trusted adult if they are unsure about a new tip they read.

Teaching them critical thinking can prevent mishaps and keep them safe.

## 21. Involving the Child in Self-Care

For small tasks like applying oil to dry skin, let the child help if they are old enough. This builds independence:

1. **Show and Tell:** Demonstrate how much oil to use, explaining that just a little dab is enough.
2. **Mirror Method:** They can stand in front of a mirror to see what they are doing, like rubbing a dry patch on their arm.
3. **Praise Their Effort:** Encourage them when they remember to care for their own skin.

This can create a positive link to simple wellness habits, making them more likely to continue as they grow up.

---

## 22. Castor Oil for Mild Nail Care in Kids

Some children have brittle nails or dry cuticles from constant handwashing or biting their nails. A dab of castor oil can keep the cuticle area soft:

1. **After Bath:** Nails and cuticles are softer.
2. **Tiny Drop:** Place a small spot of castor oil on the cuticle, massaging gently around the nail base.
3. **Reduce Biting Triggers:** If the child bites nails due to stress, castor oil might not stop the habit by itself, but it can support healthier nail growth if they are trying to quit.

---

## 23. Putting Castor Oil Away: Avoid Confusion with Other Products

In a busy household, items can get mixed up. Always store castor oil in a clearly marked bottle. Do not keep it next to cooking oils in the kitchen, to avoid accidental use in food (since not all castor oils are food-grade, and kids might mix them up). If you have multiple children, consider labeling each one's personal care items so they do not accidentally share or misuse them.

## 24. Gratitude for Simple Helpers

While we must stay mindful of safety, many parents are glad to have a few basic items at home that can serve multiple small roles. Castor oil is one such product. It does not fix everything, but it can handle a range of minor problems, from dry skin to mild hair care concerns. By respecting its limits and using it wisely, families can keep a bottle on hand for times when a gentle approach might help.

---

## 25. Conclusion of Chapter 13

Parents often look for natural items that can be used in safe, simple ways for their children. Castor oil, when applied externally in small amounts, can fit into that plan for minor skin dryness, gentle massages, or quick comfort measures like foot rubs and homemade balms. Children can also learn early how to take care of themselves in little ways, building a good foundation for future habits.

Still, keep in mind that serious symptoms or repeated problems need professional evaluation. Castor oil does not replace doctor visits for big concerns. By mixing easy home remedies with common sense and proper care, you can add castor oil to your household routine in a safe manner. It can offer mild support for daily bumps and dryness, as long as you remember to use it carefully, watch for reactions, and involve a qualified worker when in doubt.

---

# CHAPTER 14: PET AND ANIMAL USES

Castor oil is often discussed in relation to humans, but some people also wonder if it can help pets and farm animals. While animals have different bodies and needs, there may be certain safe ways to use castor oil externally on pets. However, it is important to note that not all animals react the same, and mistakes can lead to discomfort or harm. In this chapter, we will explore potential uses of castor oil for common pets like dogs and cats, as well as for other animals, and we will highlight the crucial need for caution. Always remember that a veterinarian's advice is necessary for serious issues or if you are unsure.

## 1. General Warnings for Using Castor Oil on Animals

Animals cannot speak to tell us if something stings or feels uncomfortable. Plus, some species can be more sensitive to certain substances. Keep these points in mind:

1. **No Oral Use Without Vet Approval:** Giving castor oil by mouth to animals can lead to diarrhea, dehydration, or worse. Do not add it to their food or water unless a vet specifically says it is safe in a certain dose.
2. **Avoid Raw Castor Beans:** Just like for people, raw seeds are dangerous for animals.
3. **Consider Species Differences:** What might be okay for a dog may be risky for a cat. Cats in particular can have strong reactions to certain oils.
4. **Check for Allergies:** If you apply castor oil to your pet's skin, watch for signs of irritation or increased licking of the area.
5. **Stop if Problems Arise:** If the animal seems distressed, pulls away, or develops redness, stop using castor oil and clean the area with mild soap and water if it is safe to do so.

## 2. Possible External Uses for Dogs

Dogs often deal with itchy skin, small hot spots, or dryness around the paws. Some dog owners consider castor oil for these issues:

1. **Dry Paw Pads:**
   - After a walk or bath, check the dog's paw pads.
   - If they look cracked or very dry, you can dab a tiny bit of castor oil on them.
   - Rub gently so it soaks in. Wipe off any excess to avoid slipping on floors.
2. **Small Dry Patches:**
   - If your dog has a patch of flaky skin, you could try a small dab of castor oil.
   - Keep the dog from licking the area until the oil soaks in. You might distract the dog with a treat or toy.
3. **Hot Spots:**
   - These are areas where a dog has licked or scratched, causing redness or hair loss. A vet visit is often best for hot spots. But if it is mild, and the vet agrees, you might apply a thin layer of castor oil to help keep the area from drying out.
   - Monitor carefully, because the dog's licking can worsen the spot. Sometimes a cone or protective collar is needed.

---

## 3. Cats and Their Sensitivities

Cats have unique liver and metabolic paths. Some substances safe for dogs are not safe for cats. Cats also groom themselves often, so if you put castor oil on a cat's fur or skin, they might lick it off:

1. **Avoid Large Areas:** Applying castor oil to a big portion of a cat's body can lead to the cat ingesting too much oil by grooming.
2. **Tiny, Local Use Only:** If there is a small dry patch or mild irritation (and the vet says it is okay), you can dab a minuscule amount on that spot. Watch to see if the cat tries to lick it.

3. **No Forced Oral Use:** Cat digestive systems can be upset by castor oil. Do not mix it in food or feed it directly without explicit vet approval.

Because cats are so sensitive, many owners choose other cat-safe products recommended by vets, rather than castor oil. It is better to be cautious since a cat's grooming habit means they may swallow anything on their fur.

---

## 4. Horses and Farm Animals

Farmers sometimes use castor oil on livestock in certain situations, mostly externally:

1. **Hoof Care for Horses:**
    - Some horse keepers say a little castor oil on the hooves can help keep them from drying or cracking in certain weather.
    - Only do this if you are sure it will not make the hooves too slippery or attract debris.
2. **Skin Rub for Livestock:**
    - Sheep, goats, or cows might get small patches of dryness or minor irritations.
    - A slight application of castor oil might soften the spot. But if it is a large area or a serious skin issue, a vet's input is needed.

Animals on farms have varied routines. Ensure that adding castor oil does not affect traction (for horses) or general well-being. Also, watch for dirt sticking to oiled areas, as this can worsen problems.

---

## 5. Grooming Sessions

Some owners use castor oil sparingly during grooming:

1. **For Dogs with Thick Fur:** A couple of drops rubbed between your palms might help you smooth the fur after brushing, adding shine.

But do not go near the skin in big amounts. And remember that too much oil can cause a greasy look or get on the furniture.
2. **For Horses:** After a thorough grooming, a bit of oil on a cloth might give the coat a shine in certain show settings. But talk to an experienced trainer or vet first to ensure it is acceptable.
3. **For Cats:** Grooming with oil is tricky because cats groom themselves. It is usually not suggested except on vet advice.

## 6. Minor Cuts or Scrapes

If an animal gets a small scrape (not deep or infected), some owners might consider a thin layer of castor oil after cleaning the area. The idea is to keep the spot soft, reducing cracking. However:

- **Clean First:** Use a vet-approved antiseptic or mild wash.
- **Assess the Wound:** If it is more than a surface scratch, or if there is bleeding, see a vet.
- **Watch the Animal:** Keep them from licking or rubbing it off. You may need a bandage or collar.

## 7. Repelling Some Insects?

There are stories that castor oil might help repel certain insects on animals. However, it is not a proven flea or tick remedy. It is thick, so it may catch some dirt and could irritate the animal if applied widely. For pest control, veterinary-approved products are safer and more effective. Avoid do-it-yourself approaches for fleas and ticks unless a vet says it is okay, as these pests can cause serious health issues.

## 8. No Replacement for Medications

Castor oil should not replace necessary pet medications or treatments. If a pet has a skin condition like mange, ringworm, or a severe infection, castor oil alone is not enough. Infections often need prescription creams or oral medicines. Delaying proper treatment can harm the animal. Use castor oil, if at all, only as a minor help for mild dryness or small spots, and always watch for changes.

## 9. External Massage for Sore Muscles (Dogs or Horses)

Some dogs do sports (like agility) or long runs with their owners. Horses can have muscle aches from riding or working. A short, gentle massage with a small bit of castor oil might help with stiffness:

1. **Dog Massage:**
    - Focus on large muscle groups, like the shoulders or thighs.
    - Use light pressure. Do not push deep, as dogs may find it uncomfortable.
    - Keep it brief—maybe a few minutes.
2. **Horse Massage:**
    - Horse masseurs sometimes use different oils. Castor oil could be one option, but do so only if you are experienced or have guidance.
    - Large areas of a horse's body would require significant oil, so be sure it does not become messy or cause the horse distress.

Animals often appreciate gentle touch, but it is wise to learn basic techniques from a pro or vet before attempting an extensive massage routine.

## 10. Checking Pet Reaction

Every pet is unique. Some might not mind the smell or feel of castor oil, while others might be bothered:

1. **Start Slowly:** Test a tiny spot. Wait a day. See if the pet licks it a lot, shows signs of irritation, or tries to avoid you when you bring it out.

2. **Look at Skin:** If there is redness or hair loss, discontinue use.
3. **Watch Behavior:** If the pet seems anxious or upset, do not force it.

Remember that even if castor oil is safe for humans, animals have different responses.

## 11. Avoiding Stains and Slips

If you are using castor oil on an animal indoors, place an old towel or mat under them. Oil can drip onto floors or carpets, making it slippery or leaving stains. For bigger animals like horses, you might be in a stable area anyway. But be mindful of where the oil could end up, especially if the animal shakes or moves suddenly.

## 12. Farm Use: Machinery and Tools?

Interestingly, some older farmers might have used castor oil for lubricating small parts on farm tools. This is not a pet use, but it highlights castor oil's broader uses around animals. Still, modern lubricants are often more practical for large machinery. Only mention this if you are into very traditional methods and keep it far from feed or places animals could lick it.

## 13. Potential for Easing Mild Swelling in Animals?

Some anecdotal remarks suggest that castor oil rubbed on minor swollen areas might help. For instance, if a dog or horse has a small area of puffiness from a minor bruise. However, swelling can be a sign of deeper injury. If you suspect a sprain, infection, or anything beyond a surface bruise, a vet check is best. Castor oil might reduce dryness on the surface, but it will not solve underlying trauma.

## 14. Homemade Pet Balm with Castor Oil?

A few owners like to create a natural paw or nose balm for dogs. A typical recipe might include:

- 1 tablespoon castor oil
- 1 tablespoon coconut oil
- 1 tablespoon beeswax

Melt the beeswax, then stir in the oils. Let it cool in a small tin. This can be dabbed on dog paw pads or a dry nose tip. But be sure the dog does not lick it off too much. Also, watch that you do not block the nose's breathing area. Use lightly and avoid frequent reapplication if the dog shows any dislike.

---

## 15. Rodents and Small Animals

For small pets like hamsters, guinea pigs, or rabbits, applying castor oil can be tricky. They groom themselves a lot, and any oil on the fur might be swallowed. Their digestive systems are sensitive. If they have a skin problem, it is safer to see a small animal vet who can recommend a product tested for that species. Using castor oil at home might do more harm than good in these tiny creatures.

---

## 16. Birds: High Risk

Birds have delicate systems and specialized feathers. An oil that is too heavy or unsafe can harm their ability to fly, regulate temperature, or maintain feather structure. Unless you are an avian specialist or vet, do not apply castor oil to a bird's feathers or skin. If a bird has a problem, professional care is needed. Birds groom with their beaks, so any substance on their feathers is likely to be ingested.

---

## 17. Exotic Animals

Reptiles, amphibians, and other exotic pets have unique needs. Their skin or scales may not handle castor oil well. It can block pores, trap dirt, or cause stress. Always consult a specialized vet for these animals. It is best to avoid experimenting with castor oil unless a professional confirms it is safe.

---

## 18. Barn Cats and Feral Cats

Farm owners sometimes want to help barn cats with dryness or small issues. However, as mentioned, cats are tricky with oils. They groom themselves often, and you have limited control over how much they lick. If a barn cat has a skin problem, it might be better to contact a vet or a local rescue group for safer treatments. A little castor oil on a cat's paw pads might be okay if they are cracked, but you must keep an eye on whether the cat licks it off.

---

## 19. Recognizing When to Seek a Vet

Just like with humans, mild dryness or a small patch of flaky skin can often be handled with simple measures. But animals cannot explain pain, so watch for:

- **Constant Scratching or Biting:** Could be mites, fleas, allergies, or infection. Castor oil will not fix these.
- **Large Areas of Hair Loss:** Possibly fungal or hormonal issues. Needs vet attention.
- **Oozing or Foul Smells:** Sign of infection that requires medical treatment.
- **Behavioral Changes:** If the pet becomes lethargic, loses appetite, or hides more often, it might be more serious.

Never let castor oil become a reason to skip or delay professional care.

## 20. Observing the Results Over Time

If you do try a small external application with vet support or on a mild condition, track:

- **Skin Improvement or Not:** Does the dryness get better? Or does it stay the same or worsen?
- **Licking or Scratching:** Has it increased or decreased since using the oil?
- **Frequency of Use:** Note how often you apply it, and how the animal reacts each time.

If you see no real benefit or if problems arise, stop and reconsider your approach.

---

## 21. Keeping Castor Oil Secure and Labeled

Animals might knock things over or chew on bottles if curious. Keep your castor oil bottle in a cabinet or shelf away from pets. If you have a large dog, store it where they cannot reach. Also, label the bottle "Castor Oil – For External Use" so no one accidentally uses it in a way that could harm the pet.

---

## 22. Potential Use in Insect Stings on Livestock

Farm animals can get insect stings, but they cannot complain the way humans do. Sometimes a small dab of castor oil is used on livestock stings or bites if it is a mild spot. If you see swelling, ensure it is not serious. Watch for signs of an allergic reaction. In large livestock, a vet might provide anti-inflammatory medicine if needed. Castor oil can only do so much as a surface aid.

## 23. Sheep Shearing or Goat Grooming

Some farmers rub minimal amounts of oil on shears or tools to reduce friction, but that is different from applying it to the animal. If you choose to apply a tiny amount to a goat's or sheep's dry patch, keep it minimal to avoid collecting dirt or causing the animal to fuss. Always consider how the fleece or coat might trap oil, and whether it might lead to matting or odor.

---

## 24. Thinking Twice About Home Remedies for Animals

There are many home remedy tips for pets online. While some are harmless, others can be unsafe. Castor oil is not the most dangerous item, but it can still cause trouble if misused. The best approach is to be cautious, do a little test if you are confident, and always keep an open line with a vet. If the vet suggests a commercial product, it might be specifically created and tested for that species, lowering the risk.

# CHAPTER 15: EXTERNAL THERAPIES (PACKS AND RUBBING METHODS)

Castor oil is famous for external methods that involve placing it on the skin in different ways. Many people discover that castor oil packs and rubbing methods can bring simple comfort to areas of the body that feel tight or stressed. These techniques often revolve around warming the oil, applying it to a cloth, and then keeping it in place for a certain amount of time. Others involve directly massaging the oil into the skin with gentle motions. In this chapter, we will look at the range of external castor oil therapies, why people use them, and how to perform them safely. By the end, you should know many ways to create and apply castor oil packs, as well as various rubbing methods, so that you can pick the one that best fits your needs.

## 1. What Are External Therapies?

When we say "external therapies," we mean any way that castor oil is placed on the outside of the body, instead of being swallowed. This can include:

1. **Castor Oil Pack:** A piece of cloth soaked in castor oil, often warmed, and then put on the skin.
2. **Rub or Massage:** Rubbing castor oil with the hands directly onto a part of the body.
3. **Warm Compresses with Castor Oil:** Using a warmed towel or wrap on top of an area where castor oil has been applied.

Each method has its own purpose. Some people like the packs for deeper, slower support. Others prefer a quick rub or gentle massage when they only have a few minutes. The main point is to let the castor oil rest on the skin so that the body can enjoy the soothing feel and any benefits linked to the oil's unique parts.

## 2. Why People Choose External Methods

There are a few reasons many turn to external castor oil therapies:

- **Simple to Do at Home:** You only need cloths, towels, and castor oil.
- **Targeted Approach:** You can place the oil exactly where you want it, such as on the abdomen or on a stiff joint.
- **Less Risk than Swallowing:** External use generally has fewer side effects, because you are not consuming the oil in large amounts.
- **Relaxing Routine:** Many enjoy the process of lying down with a warm pack or taking a few minutes for a small self-massage. It can be a break from a busy day.

## 3. Basic Supplies for Castor Oil Packs and Rubs

Before we get into the methods, gather the supplies you need:

1. **Castor Oil:** High-quality, cold-pressed oil is often preferred. You can still use other kinds if that is what you have.
2. **Cloth or Flannel:** This should be clean and able to hold oil without falling apart. Many people use cotton or wool flannel.
3. **Plastic Wrap or Towel:** You might put plastic wrap or a towel on top of the oil-soaked cloth to keep it from making a mess.
4. **Heating Pad or Hot Water Bottle (Optional):** This can help warm the pack once it is on your body. Make sure the heat is not too high.
5. **Old Towel or Sheet:** You might place this under you to catch any drips or spills.
6. **Soap and Water:** For clean-up afterward, since castor oil is thick and can be sticky.

For rubbing or massage, you mainly need your hands, the oil, and possibly a towel to wipe off extra oil. Some people also have a small bowl of warm water nearby to keep their hands at a comfortable temperature.

## 4. Making a Castor Oil Pack

The most common external therapy people talk about is the castor oil pack. Here is how you can make and apply one:

**Step 1: Cut or Fold the Cloth**
Pick a piece of cloth that will fit the area you want to cover. If you are targeting your abdomen, measure enough cloth to cover that region. If you are focusing on a knee or elbow, you will need a smaller piece. Fold it so that it has a few layers, helping hold more oil.

**Step 2: Warm the Oil (Optional)**
Some prefer to warm the castor oil a bit before soaking the cloth. You can do this by placing the oil bottle in a bowl of warm water. Do not make it too hot. It should be just above body temperature.

**Step 3: Soak the Cloth**
Pour enough castor oil onto the cloth so that the fabric is well-saturated, but not dripping. You can also put the cloth in a shallow dish and drizzle oil on it, pressing it gently to help the oil spread evenly.

**Step 4: Placement**
Lie down or sit in a comfortable position. Place the soaked cloth on the target area (for example, your stomach or a sore joint). Make sure it lies smoothly against your skin, with no big wrinkles.

**Step 5: Cover It**
To keep the oil from staining clothes or furniture, place a piece of plastic wrap or an old towel on top of the cloth. Many people then add a heating pad on low or medium heat for extra warmth. If you do not have a heating pad, you can use a hot water bottle. Just be sure it is not so hot that it burns your skin.

**Step 6: Relax**
Most individuals keep the castor oil pack on for 20 to 60 minutes. You can read a book, listen to calming music, or just close your eyes. This is a good chance to rest.

**Step 7: Clean Up**
When you are done, remove the cloth. You can store it in a sealed bag if you want to use it again. Wipe off any extra oil on your skin with paper towels or wash it off with mild soap and warm water.

## 5. Using a Castor Oil Pack on the Abdomen

One popular spot for castor oil packs is the abdomen. People often say this helps with mild digestive issues or general relaxation. Here are a few tips:

1. **Target Area:** You can place it over the upper right side to focus on the liver region. Or you can place it more centrally if your goal is general stomach comfort.
2. **Timing:** Many like to do this at night before sleep. They say it helps them unwind. Others do it during the day if they have time.
3. **Frequency:** Some do it two or three times a week. Others only once a month. It depends on what feels best for you.

## 6. Pack for Joints or Muscles

If you have a tight knee, sore elbow, or a stiff shoulder, you can still use a castor oil pack:

1. **Adjust the Cloth Size:** Cut a piece of cloth that will wrap around the joint easily.
2. **Gentle Movement:** Before placing the pack, you might do a small range-of-motion movement to loosen the area.
3. **Wrap Carefully:** You can secure the pack with plastic wrap or a bandage, but do not wrap it so tightly that you restrict blood flow.

4. **Shorter Sessions:** Sometimes joints feel better after 20 minutes rather than an hour. Pay attention to how it feels.

---

# 7. Reusing Your Pack

Some people reuse the same cloth for their castor oil packs. After the session, they fold the oil-soaked cloth and put it in a sealed container or plastic bag in the fridge. Others prefer a fresh cloth each time to avoid any risk of dirt or bacteria building up. If you do reuse the cloth, watch for any unpleasant smell or discoloration that might mean it is time to discard it and use a new one.

---

# 8. The Massage or Rubbing Method

Beyond packs, you can simply rub castor oil into your skin in certain areas. This can be:

1. **Quick Daily Spot Treatment:** For example, rubbing a bit of oil on your elbows, knees, or hands if they are dry.
2. **Larger Muscle Massage:** For sore muscles, some do a gentle full massage. They might blend castor oil with a lighter oil like grape seed oil to help it spread.
3. **Foot Rub at Night:** A small foot rub with castor oil before bed can help keep the feet from cracking and might feel soothing after standing or walking all day.

The advantage of this method is that it is faster than making a pack. You do not need cloths or plastic wrap. But it might not provide as deep of a warming effect unless you also add a warm compress or do a more thorough rub.

## 9. Adding Mild Heat to a Rub

If you prefer to rub castor oil directly onto the skin but still want warmth, you have options:

- **Use Warm Water:** Before starting, soak your hands in warm water or run them under warm water. Dry them, and then pour some castor oil into your palms. The warmth in your hands will help the oil feel more comfortable.
- **Warm Towel Compress:** After rubbing the oil onto, say, your shoulder or thigh, drape a warm, damp towel on top for a few minutes. Renew the towel's warmth as needed.

This mild heat can relax muscles and might help the skin absorb the oil a bit better.

---

## 10. Castor Oil in Bath Water?

Because castor oil is thick, it does not blend well with water. If you place it directly in the tub, it might float in small drops or stick to the tub's surface, making it slippery. Some people try to mix castor oil with Epsom salts or mild liquid soap first, so it disperses more evenly. Even then, you have to be careful because the tub can become slick. If you want an "oil bath" feeling, it might be easier to use a lighter oil. However, if you are careful and do not mind cleaning up, you can still attempt a small amount of castor oil in a warm bath.

---

## 11. Face Packs and Masks

Some individuals like to do a mini castor oil pack or rub for the face, but caution is important:

1. **Small Sections:** A large cloth pack on the face can be messy. Instead, you can soak a small piece of cloth or cotton pad with a tiny bit of oil, placing it on a dry patch or an area you want to treat.

2. **Avoid Eyes and Mouth:** The thick oil can irritate eyes or feel unpleasant if it drips near the mouth.
3. **Short Time:** The skin on the face can be sensitive. Some do 10-15 minutes max, then rinse with warm water.

If you have acne or are prone to breakouts, test a small patch first. Castor oil can clog pores for some people.

---

## 12. Scalp and Hair Packs

Chapter 6 covered hair care with castor oil, but you can also do a "scalp pack" by soaking a cloth in warm oil and placing it on your scalp. This can be tricky:

1. **Protect Your Clothes and Furniture:** Oil can drip down the sides of your face and onto the floor or fabric.
2. **Cover with a Shower Cap:** This can trap the heat and keep the oil from running everywhere.
3. **Time Limit:** About 20-30 minutes is often enough. Afterward, wash thoroughly. You might need two rounds of shampoo.

This method can help a dry scalp or hair strands in need of deeper moisture, but prepare for the clean-up.

---

## 13. Gentle Movements During a Pack Session

If your aim is relaxation, you can lie still with your pack. But if you want mild support for a joint or muscle, some suggest doing small, easy movements while the pack is in place or during short breaks:

- **Slow Knee Bends:** If the pack is on your knee, try gently bending and straightening your leg a few times after it has been in place for 10 minutes.
- **Shoulder Rolls:** If your shoulder has the pack, do careful rotations to keep it from stiffening.

Keep the movements mild so you do not shift the pack too much. The idea is to pair warmth with gentle mobility.

## 14. Dealing with Leaks and Spills

Castor oil is thick and can stain. Here are some tips to avoid big messes:

1. **Use Old Towels or Sheets:** Do not use your favorite bed sheets. Have a dedicated "castor oil towel" and a place where you lie down for the session.
2. **Check the Cloth Edges:** Make sure the oil is not dripping from the sides of the cloth. If it is, dab away extra oil or fold the cloth so it is not saturated at the edges.
3. **Keep a Wipe Nearby:** Paper towels or old rags can help you quickly wipe up any drips.

## 15. Oils to Mix with Castor Oil for Rubbing

If you find castor oil too thick, you can blend it with other oils:

- **Coconut Oil (Fractionated):** This remains liquid at room temperature, which can thin out castor oil.
- **Olive Oil:** Common in kitchens, can make the mixture easier to spread.
- **Almond Oil:** Has a mild smell and is often used in massage blends.

A 1:1 ratio (half castor oil, half another oil) is a common starting point. Adjust as needed until you like the feel.

## 16. Short vs. Long Sessions

How long you keep a castor oil pack on or how long you rub the oil can vary:

- **Short Session (10-20 minutes):** Good if you are in a hurry, or if you are trying it for the first time and want to see how your body responds.
- **Long Session (30-60 minutes):** For deeper relaxation or if you are targeting a specific area that feels quite stiff. Some do it for up to an hour, especially the abdomen or certain muscle groups.
- **Overnight:** A few individuals wrap a castor oil pack and go to sleep with it. This can be messy, so they wear old clothes or protect the bedding well. It might be too long for some people, so proceed with caution if you plan to sleep with the pack.

## 17. Who Might Benefit from External Therapies?

A range of people use these methods. For example:

1. **Office Workers:** Those who sit for long hours might get stiff backs or shoulders. A castor oil rub or pack can offer some ease in the evening.
2. **Physically Active Individuals:** Runners or laborers might find relief from muscle tightness or mild soreness.
3. **Folks with Mild Digestion Woes:** Some use the abdominal pack to feel calmer, though it is not a cure for digestive issues.
4. **Stress Relief Seekers:** The routine of applying a warm pack, lying down, and taking a moment for yourself can help reduce tension mentally, too.

## 18. Do's and Don'ts of External Methods

Do's:

- **Do Test on a Small Patch:** If you have never used castor oil externally, apply a tiny amount on your forearm to check for any reaction.
- **Do Use Gentle Heat:** Warmth can help, but do not burn yourself. Medium or low settings on a heating pad are usually enough.

- **Do Stay Hydrated:** This can be helpful if your body is relaxing or if you are trying to support normal bodily functions.

**Don'ts:**

- **Don't Rub Too Hard:** If you massage vigorously with thick oil, you can irritate your skin. Use moderate pressure.
- **Don't Overuse:** Daily packs for extended periods might lead to skin dryness or other issues. Listen to your body.
- **Don't Ignore Pain:** If you experience sharp pain or big changes in the area, stop and see a professional.

## 19. Timing with Your Daily Schedule

Deciding when to do an external therapy depends on your lifestyle:

- **Morning Use:** Some like a quick rub on stiff joints after waking up, to help them move better.
- **Midday Break:** If you work from home or have free time, you could do a 20-minute pack on your lunch break.
- **Evening Wind-Down:** Many prefer castor oil packs at night to relax. They might watch a quiet show or read while the pack is on.

Pick a slot when you can be still and not be rushed. The experience is more pleasant if you can focus on calmness rather than chores.

## 20. Reaching Hard-to-Access Spots

It can be tricky to put a castor oil pack on your own back or shoulders. You may need help from a friend or family member. For a shoulder, you might be able to do it yourself if you place a cloth on a chair, soak it in oil, and then lean back onto it carefully. Just be sure you do not accidentally slide off or let the cloth slip away. Some folks drape plastic wrap or an old T-shirt on the back of a chair, add the oil, and then lean into it so it touches the shoulder blade area.

## 21. Special Notes for Sensitive Skin

If you have sensitive skin or a history of reactions, be extra careful:

1. **Shorter Time First:** Maybe only 10 minutes to start.
2. **No Additional Heat Right Away:** The combination of oil and heat can intensify effects. Start without heat.
3. **Avoid Large Areas:** Focus on a small patch or single spot before moving to bigger areas.

If you notice a rash, itching, or redness, wash the area, discontinue use, and keep an eye on your skin. If it does not get better soon, you might want to talk to a health professional.

## 22. What to Expect After an External Session

After removing a castor oil pack or finishing a rub:

- **Skin Might Feel Oily:** You can blot off extra oil with an old cloth or paper towel, then wash with mild soap if you wish.
- **Area May Feel Warmer or Looser:** Some people report a warm, relaxed feeling in the targeted area.
- **Possible Calm Mood:** The restful process might lead to feeling a bit sleepy or serene.

If you feel irritation or dryness, it could mean your skin is sensitive or you left the pack on too long. Adjust the session next time.

## 23. Pairing External Therapies with Other Steps

External castor oil methods can go hand in hand with other mild steps:

- **Stretching:** Do a gentle stretch routine before or after.

- **Herbal Teas or Water:** Some folks sip herbal tea to stay calm and hydrated.
- **Light Meditation:** Deep breathing can help the mind settle while the body rests under a warm pack.
- **Comfortable Lighting:** Dim lights or relaxing music can boost the soothing atmosphere.

Combining a few small changes can turn a simple pack or rub into a short wellness break in your day.

---

## 24. Kids and External Therapies

We covered this in Chapter 13 in detail, but to summarize:

- **Child-Friendly Approach:** If you use a castor oil pack on a child's abdomen for mild tummy issues, do it for a shorter time, such as 10-15 minutes.
- **Monitor Closely:** Children might not speak up if it feels too hot or uncomfortable. Check in often.
- **Avoid Large Amounts:** Keep the cloth from being soaking wet with oil, and do not do very long sessions with kids.

Always be extra careful with heat around children.

# CHAPTER 16: SAFETY MEASURES AND WARNINGS

Castor oil has a long history of use, both inside and outside the body. While many people have good experiences, it is still important to know the possible risks. The fact that something is "natural" does not mean it is always free of concerns. In this chapter, we will talk about safety rules, warnings, and the steps you can take to avoid problems when using castor oil. From choosing the right type of oil to recognizing signs of allergic reactions, you will find guidance here to help you feel secure in your decisions about castor oil.

## 1. Why Safety Rules Matter

Castor oil can be powerful. Used correctly, it can help with dryness or mild digestive needs. Used incorrectly, it may cause discomfort like cramps, skin rash, or dehydration. By learning basic safety rules, you reduce the chance of trouble. This is especially important if you are dealing with children, older adults, or pets. We will look at each topic so that you know what to do, what not to do, and when to ask for professional help.

## 2. Possible Side Effects

Even though castor oil is generally safe for many people when used responsibly, side effects can appear:

1. **Skin Irritation:** Redness, itching, or a rash can happen if someone's skin is sensitive or if the oil is left on for too long.
2. **Allergic Reaction:** Though rare, some folks might have an allergy to components in castor oil. This can lead to more severe symptoms, including swelling or hives.

3. **Digestive Trouble (When Taken Internally):** If you swallow castor oil, you might feel cramps, diarrhea, or an urgent need to go to the bathroom. Overuse can cause dehydration and electrolyte imbalance.
4. **Nausea or Vomiting:** The thick taste or strong effect on the gut can trigger these, especially if you take too much.

Recognizing these signs early helps you respond quickly, whether that means rinsing the skin, drinking fluids, or seeking medical advice.

---

## 3. The Risk of Toxic Seeds

Raw castor seeds contain a dangerous protein called ricin. This substance can be extremely harmful. During the manufacturing process for castor oil, the seeds are pressed in ways that remove or destroy ricin. As a result, properly made castor oil should not have harmful levels of ricin. However, it is crucial not to eat raw castor beans or seeds. If you ever see them in the wild, avoid them, and keep children away as well. Castor oil sold for health or beauty use is processed to remove these dangers.

---

## 4. Picking the Right Kind of Castor Oil

When shopping for castor oil, you might see several labels:

- **Cold-Pressed:** Generally made without high heat, which might keep more of the oil's original structure intact.
- **Expeller-Pressed:** Made with some mechanical pressure, possibly generating some heat from friction.
- **Refined or Deodorized:** The oil may have been filtered or heated to remove odors and impurities.
- **Black Castor Oil:** Often associated with Jamaican black castor oil, which has a darker color due to roasting the seeds.

Each type can be safe if produced correctly. Check that the oil is labeled for the use you have in mind. If you want to swallow castor oil, look for food-grade or one specifically labeled as safe for internal use. Some castor oils are labeled for external use only.

## 5. Allergy Testing

Because allergies can happen, it is wise to do a patch test if you plan to use castor oil on your skin or hair, especially if you have never used it before. Here is how:

1. **Pick a Small Spot:** The inside of your forearm is a good area.
2. **Apply a Drop:** Rub it in gently and let it sit.
3. **Wait 24 Hours:** Watch for any redness, itchiness, or swelling.
4. **Check for Changes:** If you see nothing unusual, you are likely safe to use it on a larger area.

If you notice itching or redness, wash it off. Do not continue using castor oil without talking to a health professional if you see a reaction.

## 6. Safe Internal Use: Dos and Don'ts

Some people choose to swallow castor oil for occasional constipation or other reasons. If you plan to do this, keep these rules in mind:

1. **Speak with a Professional:** If you have medical conditions or take other medicines, talk to a doctor or pharmacist before using castor oil internally.
2. **Measure Carefully:** Follow guidelines on the bottle or from a health professional. Typical adult dosages might range from 1 teaspoon to 1 tablespoon.
3. **Know Potential Effects:** Castor oil can work fast. You may need to stay near a bathroom for several hours.
4. **Stay Hydrated:** Because it can increase bowel movements, drink extra water to avoid dehydration.
5. **Do Not Overdo It:** Regular or heavy use can lead to cramps, diarrhea, and an upset balance in the gut.

If you find yourself needing castor oil often for constipation, see a health professional. There might be a better plan for your digestive health.

## 7. Swallowing Castor Oil During Pregnancy

Many have heard the old advice that pregnant people can use castor oil to "start labor." However, using castor oil internally in pregnancy can cause strong contractions and discomfort. Without the oversight of a doctor or midwife, this is not recommended. It can pose risks to both parent and baby if done without guidance. If you are pregnant and thinking about castor oil, speak to a healthcare worker who can explain the pros and cons based on your specific situation.

## 8. Safe Temperatures for Warm Packs

A common external use is the warm castor oil pack. Remember:

1. **Check the Heat:** Use your wrist or the inside of your forearm to see if it feels comfortable. If it is too hot for your skin, it could burn you.
2. **Be Aware of Layers:** If you have multiple layers (cloth, plastic wrap, heating pad), it can trap more heat. Check occasionally so it does not get too warm.
3. **Shorter Sessions for Sensitive Skin:** If you have very sensitive skin, keep the heat mild, or skip the heat and just let the oil do its work at room temperature.

## 9. Handling and Storing Castor Oil

Because castor oil can degrade or change quality if exposed to heat or light for too long, store it properly:

1. **Cool, Dark Spot:** A cupboard away from sunlight is good.

2. **Tightly Sealed:** Air entering the bottle can speed up spoilage or contamination.
3. **Watch the Date:** Some bottles have a recommended use-by date. If the oil smells rancid or shows a change in color, it might be time to replace it.

Keeping it away from children or pets is also wise, so they do not accidentally spill or swallow it.

---

## 10. Avoiding Eye Contact

Some people use castor oil near their eyelashes or eyebrows. While a tiny amount is often okay if it is a high-quality oil, you should avoid getting it in your eyes. The thickness can blur your vision or irritate the surface of the eye. If it does happen, rinse gently with water or eye drops. If irritation remains, seek help from an eye care professional.

---

## 11. Concerns About Pore Clogging

While castor oil can be good for dryness, some individuals find it too heavy. People whose skin clogs easily might develop pimples if they use a lot of castor oil on their face or scalp. If you are prone to breakouts, try a small test area on the face, or dilute the castor oil with a lighter oil. Stop if you see a surge in clogged pores.

---

## 12. Frequency of Use

Moderation is key with castor oil:

- **External Use:** Many do not need daily castor oil packs or rubs. Two or three times a week might be enough for mild dryness or stiffness.

- **Internal Use:** Frequent internal use can lead to dependence or digestive upset. Experts usually suggest occasional use at most, unless a professional instructs otherwise.
- **Children and Animals:** Use it sparingly and only when you are sure it is safe.

If you see no improvement or if the problem persists, a professional's advice is likely the better approach.

---

## 13. Combining Castor Oil with Other Substances

Some people blend castor oil with herbs, essential oils, or other natural items. This can be fine, but watch for:

1. **Double Allergies:** If you add an essential oil, you might introduce a new allergen. Test it first.
2. **Strength of Essential Oils:** These can be powerful. Use only a few drops per tablespoon of castor oil.
3. **Stinging or Burning:** Certain items like strong spices (ginger, for instance) can irritate skin if combined incorrectly.

Always do a small patch test when mixing new items.

---

## 14. Pets and Wildlife

We covered in Chapter 14 how to use castor oil for animals, but repeating the key point: do not leave castor oil within reach of curious pets. They can knock it over or lick it up, leading to stomach trouble. If you use castor oil on an animal, keep an eye on them and check for reactions. If they act strangely or show signs of discomfort, see a vet.

## 15. Potential Risks for Older Adults

Older adults can be more sensitive to changes in bowel habits or skin dryness. Taking castor oil by mouth for older adults might lead to dehydration or low potassium levels if they have diarrhea. If you are older or caring for someone older, start with small amounts, ensure good fluid intake, and watch for any weakness or dizziness. For external use, watch the skin for dryness or tears.

---

## 16. Interactions with Medicines

Any strong laxative or substance that moves the bowels can alter how medicines pass through the gut. If you are on prescription drugs, especially those that rely on slow absorption, castor oil might reduce how much of the drug your body takes in. Blood pressure medicines, certain heart meds, or others might be affected by ongoing diarrhea. Talk to a pharmacist or doctor about any risk. Externally, there is less concern about direct drug interaction, but it never hurts to ask if you have a condition that affects the skin or circulation.

---

## 17. Signs of Serious Trouble

While mild side effects can happen, certain signs suggest a bigger problem:

1. **Breathing Difficulty, Swelling of Lips or Tongue:** This can signal a strong allergic reaction. Seek medical help immediately.
2. **Severe Abdominal Pain or Bloody Stools:** This might mean something other than mild constipation. Stop using castor oil and get help.
3. **Fainting or Extreme Weakness:** Could be linked to dehydration or electrolyte imbalance from excessive bowel movements. Contact a health worker at once.

If any of these happen, do not wait to see if it goes away. A professional can check vital signs and guide you.

## 18. Children's Dosage and Warnings

In Chapter 13, we described how to handle castor oil with children. But it is worth repeating: giving castor oil by mouth to children can be risky. Children's bodies can lose fluids rapidly. External use also needs care—shorter time frames, mild heat, and gentle application. If you think a child might benefit from castor oil for digestion, ask a pediatrician rather than guessing.

## 19. Avoiding Prolonged Use

Some individuals try to use castor oil internally long-term for weight management or daily bowel movement control. This approach can be harmful. Over time, the bowel might depend on strong stimulation. The body might also lose electrolytes or face vitamin absorption issues. As for external use, daily large applications might dry or irritate the skin. Aim for balance. If you have a chronic condition, get a plan from a health professional.

## 20. Handling Castor Oil in Public or Shared Spaces

If you do a castor oil pack at a shared location—maybe a dorm or group home—be mindful of:

1. **Privacy:** The process can be messy. Find a private corner where you can lie down.
2. **Hygiene:** Dispose of cloths or towels properly. Clean up any spills to prevent slips or mold.
3. **Time Constraints:** If you need to do it for 30 minutes, be sure you have that time free. Rushing the process can lead to spillage and stress.

## 21. Reading Labels Carefully

Labels often show recommended uses. If a product says "For Cosmetic Use Only," it might not be food-grade. Do not swallow it. Also, check if the label warns about eye contact or if it suggests a patch test. These details often come from the maker's own testing and can guide safe use.

---

## 22. Dealing with Stains on Fabric

If castor oil gets on clothes or sheets, removing it can be challenging. You can:

1. **Blot First:** Use paper towels to lift excess oil.
2. **Pre-Treat with Dish Soap:** Rub a bit of dish soap into the stain before washing, as dish soap can cut through grease.
3. **Wash with Warm or Hot Water (Check Fabric Care):** Some materials can handle higher temperatures, which help break down oils. If the item still shows a stain, consider repeating or using a commercial stain remover.

Avoid tossing oil-soaked cloths into the dryer until the stain is gone, as heat can set the stain.

---

## 23. Expiry and Old Oil

Castor oil can go rancid after a while. The smell might become off or sour. If that happens, do not use it on your body or swallow it. While rancid oil might not always cause severe harm, it can irritate the skin and is not pleasant. If your bottle is old, you can do a sniff test. If it smells normal (mild or somewhat earthy) and you see no cloudiness or separation, it might still be okay. But trust your instincts: if it seems odd, replace it.

## 24. Common Myths About Safety

1. **"You Cannot Be Allergic to Castor Oil Because It's Natural"**: Not true. People can be allergic to many natural items.
2. **"Castor Oil Is Always Safe for Babies"**: Babies have more delicate systems. Do not use it on them internally unless a pediatrician says so. Even external use should be minimal and supervised.
3. **"You Can Drink as Much as You Want If It's Food-Grade"**: Overdosing can lead to severe diarrhea, dehydration, and an imbalance in the body.

---

## 25. Wrapping Up Safety Measures

Castor oil can be a supportive friend in the home if you follow simple guidelines. Whether you use it for a short rub on dry skin or as a once-in-a-while remedy for mild constipation, knowledge is your best defense against problems. Test for allergies, pick the right type of oil, use modest amounts, and do not ignore warnings. If you find yourself in doubt, a health worker's advice is often the surest path.

In the chapters to come, we will explore more about mixing castor oil with other oils and herbs, as well as modern research that shines light on how castor oil works. But the key lesson is this: a bit of caution goes a long way. By respecting castor oil's power and following these safety measures, you can include it in your wellness routines with more confidence.

# CHAPTER 17: MIXING WITH OTHER OILS AND HERBS

Castor oil is often used on its own, but many people also like to mix it with other oils and herbs to create blends that offer added benefits. These combinations can be applied to the skin, scalp, or hair, depending on what you want to achieve. In this chapter, we will look at how castor oil can work together with common oils such as coconut, olive, and almond, as well as selected herbs or herb-infused oils. We will cover general guidelines for mixing, what to watch out for, and how to store your mixtures. By the end, you should have an idea of how to design your own custom blends, whether you want a softer lotion, a stronger hair mask, or a gentle massage oil that has more than one function.

## 1. Why Mix Castor Oil at All?

Castor oil is quite thick and sticky on its own. Some users find it hard to spread over large areas of the body or scalp. By blending it with other liquids, you can change its texture and reduce the stickiness. In addition, different oils bring their own traits. For example, coconut oil is known to help keep skin soft, and olive oil is often praised for vitamins that can benefit the hair. By combining them, you might get a more balanced product that is easier to apply and that delivers multiple benefits.

Herbs or essential oils can also add special qualities. Some might soothe mild redness, while others give a pleasant aroma. A custom blend allows you to pick ingredients that match your goals, like calming your scalp, easing tension in muscles, or making a richer lotion. However, it is crucial to remember that each extra ingredient can raise the chance of a reaction, so you should test your final mixture before using it on a large area.

## 2. Basic Rules for Mixing Castor Oil with Other Oils

When combining castor oil with another carrier oil, consider these tips:

1. **Pick a Partner Oil:** Common choices include coconut, olive, almond, jojoba, grape seed, or argan oil. All are widely available, have mild scents, and can help make the mixture less dense.
2. **Ratios Matter:** A good starting point is a 1:1 ratio (equal parts castor oil and another oil). You can adjust from there—if the end product is still too thick, add more of the lighter oil. If it feels too runny, increase the castor oil.
3. **Blend in a Clean Container:** Use a glass or plastic bottle that has been washed and dried thoroughly. If possible, use a dark-colored container to protect the mix from light.
4. **Label the Mixture:** Write down the date and the ratio you used. This makes it easier to reproduce if you like the final product.
5. **Storage:** Keep the mixture away from heat and direct sunlight. A cool cupboard is usually fine. If you see separation, just shake the bottle gently before use.

---

## 3. Examples of Simple Oil Combinations

### A. Coconut and Castor Oil for Hair

- **Ratio:** 1 part castor oil to 1 part coconut oil.
- **Main Use:** Apply to the scalp and hair ends to help with dryness or brittleness. You can leave it on for 20-30 minutes (or even overnight, if you wear a shower cap) before washing thoroughly.
- **Note:** If you live in a cold climate, coconut oil might become solid at low temperatures. You can warm the mixture gently in a bowl of warm water.

### B. Olive and Castor Oil for Skin

- **Ratio:** 2 parts olive oil to 1 part castor oil.
- **Main Use:** Rub a small amount onto dry skin patches or rough elbows and knees. This blend is thinner than pure castor oil, so it might spread more easily.

- **Note:** Olive oil has a stronger scent, so some people add a drop or two of a mild essential oil to mask it.

### C. Almond and Castor Oil for Massage

- **Ratio:** 1 part castor oil to 2 parts almond oil.
- **Main Use:** Gentle massages on arms, legs, or back. Almond oil has a lighter consistency, so it helps the mix glide without leaving too thick of a film.
- **Note:** Almond oil can spoil if stored too long, so make a small batch if you do not use it often.

---

## 4. Adding Herbs to Your Mixture

There are two main ways to incorporate herbs:

1. **Essential Oils:** These are highly concentrated, often extracted by steam or other methods. Examples include lavender, rosemary, peppermint, and chamomile. A little goes a long way, so be cautious.
2. **Infused Oils:** You can create your own by soaking dried herbs in a carrier oil for several weeks. Once strained, the oil carries some of the plant's qualities. Alternatively, you can buy pre-made herb-infused oils.

When mixing with castor oil, remember:

- **Use a Small Amount of Essential Oil:** Typically, only 1-2 drops per tablespoon of the carrier blend. More can irritate the skin.
- **Choose Herbs that Match Your Goal:** For a soothing effect, you might pick chamomile or lavender. For a "fresh" or invigorating blend, consider rosemary or peppermint.
- **Test for Reactions:** Some essential oils can cause redness or itching. Always do a patch test.

## 5. Potential Benefits of Certain Herbs

- **Lavender:** Known for a calm scent. Some use it to support relaxation.
- **Rosemary:** Often linked to scalp care. Some believe it can help with mild scalp dryness or add a fresh smell to hair products.
- **Peppermint:** Gives a cooling sensation. Must be used in small amounts, or it can feel tingly or burn.
- **Chamomile:** Believed to help calm mild skin irritation. Usually gentle, but still do a patch test.

If you are making a castor oil pack that you want to smell nice or provide extra comfort, you can add a drop or two of these. Just be careful not to use strong herbs on sensitive areas, and avoid anything that might sting if you have cracks or open skin.

---

## 6. Practical Steps for Making an Herb-Infused Castor Oil

If you want to infuse castor oil directly with dried herbs (rather than using essential oils), here is a basic method:

1. **Choose Dried Herbs:** Examples might include dried calendula petals, dried chamomile flowers, or dried rosemary leaves. Avoid fresh herbs, because their water content can lead to mold growth.
2. **Sterilize a Jar:** Wash and dry a jar thoroughly. Some boil the jar in water for added cleanliness. Let it cool.
3. **Fill with Herbs:** Place the dried herbs in the jar, filling it about one-third of the way.
4. **Add Castor Oil:** Pour castor oil (or a castor-other-oil blend) over the herbs until they are fully covered. Leave a little space at the top.
5. **Seal and Label:** Write the date and contents on the jar.
6. **Steep:** Keep the jar in a cool, dark place for 2-6 weeks, shaking it gently every few days.
7. **Strain:** After the desired time, strain the oil through cheesecloth or a fine sieve to remove the herb bits.
8. **Use or Store:** Transfer the infused oil to a clean container. Store it away from direct sunlight.

This process allows castor oil to pick up some of the herb's properties over time. The resulting oil might smell or feel slightly different, and it can be used in the same ways as regular castor oil.

---

## 7. Common Mixes for Hair and Scalp Care

1. **Castor Oil + Jojoba Oil + Rosemary Essential Oil**
   - **Why:** Jojoba oil is similar to skin's natural oils, so it can help balance the scalp. Rosemary essential oil is often used for scalp freshness.
   - **How:** Blend 2 tablespoons castor oil, 2 tablespoons jojoba oil, and 2-3 drops rosemary oil. Massage into the scalp, wait 20 minutes, then wash out thoroughly.
2. **Castor Oil + Coconut Oil + Lavender Essential Oil**
   - **Why:** Coconut oil helps with dryness, lavender can bring a gentle scent.
   - **How:** Melt 2 tablespoons coconut oil (if solid), add 1 tablespoon castor oil, and 1-2 drops lavender. Apply to hair ends or scalp. Leave on for at least 15 minutes, then rinse.

---

## 8. Mixes for Skin Soothing

1. **Castor Oil + Olive Oil + Chamomile**
   - **Why:** Chamomile is calming, and olive oil helps spread the thick castor oil.
   - **How:** Infuse olive oil with dried chamomile for a few weeks (or buy chamomile-infused oil). Blend it 1:1 with castor oil. Use on dry elbows, knees, or mild rough patches.
2. **Castor Oil + Almond Oil + Calendula Flowers**
   - **Why:** Calendula is sometimes used for mild skin support.
   - **How:** Infuse almond oil with calendula flowers, strain, and then blend equal parts with castor oil. Rub a small amount onto chapped areas.

## 9. Making a Simple Lotion or Balm

You can combine castor oil, a lighter oil, and beeswax to create a soft balm:

1. **Ingredients:** 2 tablespoons castor oil, 2 tablespoons coconut oil or olive oil, 2 tablespoons beeswax pastilles.
2. **Melt:** In a double boiler, melt the beeswax on low heat. Stir in the other oils.
3. **Optional Extras:** Add 1-2 drops of an essential oil for scent.
4. **Pour and Cool:** Pour into a small jar or tin. Once it cools, you have a balm. Use it on feet, hands, or lips.

This balm can be adjusted by changing the ratio of beeswax to oils, depending on how firm you want it. If it is too hard, use less beeswax. If too soft, add more beeswax.

---

## 10. Potential Problems When Mixing Oils and Herbs

- **Rancidity:** Some oils spoil faster than castor oil. If you use something like flaxseed oil or unrefined oils, the shelf life may be shorter. Smell the blend regularly to ensure it has not turned bad.
- **Allergic Reactions:** Each new ingredient introduces a risk. If you add essential oils, test the final product with a patch test.
- **Separation:** Certain oils have different densities. If they separate in the bottle, shake it gently before use.
- **Herb Quality:** Using low-quality or moldy herbs can ruin your batch. Only use dried herbs that are in good condition.

---

## 11. Storing Your Castor Oil Blends

After creating a blend, place it in an airtight bottle or jar. Dark amber or cobalt blue bottles can help block out light, preserving the oils longer. Store in a cool spot, away from heat sources like stoves or direct sun. If you notice any odd smell, color change, or mold (in the case of an infusion), discard it. Natural blends typically last from a few weeks to several months, depending on the oils used.

## 12. Using a Mixture in a Castor Oil Pack

If you like using castor oil packs, you can soak your cloth in a blend instead of plain castor oil. This can bring a milder scent or specific herbal qualities:

1. **Heat with Care:** Some essential oils are sensitive to heat. High temperatures can alter their smell or break them down. Keep your heating pad on a lower setting if you are using essential oils.
2. **Avoid Irritating Herbs:** Certain herbs might irritate skin when heated. If you are uncertain, skip them or do a short test.
3. **Watch for Staining and Cleanup:** Any dyed herbs or strong-scented oils can leave deeper stains on cloths. If that matters to you, pick lighter oils and mild herbs.

## 13. Idea: A "Sleepy Time" Rub

Some people want to relax before bed. You can make a rub specifically for evening use:

- **Ingredients:** Castor oil, sweet almond oil, a few drops of lavender essential oil, and (if desired) one drop of chamomile essential oil.
- **Ratio:** 1 tablespoon castor oil, 1 tablespoon almond oil, 1-2 drops lavender, 1 drop chamomile.
- **Use:** Massage a tiny amount onto feet or shoulders before bed. The calming scent may help you feel at ease.

Remember, essential oils can be strong, so do not exceed 2-3 drops total in a tablespoon of carrier oils.

## 14. Idea: A "Refreshing" Scalp Massage Blend

For an energizing scalp massage, try:

- **Ingredients:** 1 tablespoon castor oil, 1 tablespoon grape seed oil, 1 drop peppermint essential oil, 1 drop rosemary essential oil.
- **Use:** Warm slightly, then massage into the scalp for a few minutes. The peppermint might feel cool, and the rosemary adds a fresh aroma. Rinse thoroughly afterward, so you do not leave the scalp oily.

Again, watch for any scalp irritation. Peppermint can be too strong for some people.

---

## 15. Creating a Home "Oil Bar" for Experiments

If you enjoy mixing oils regularly, you might keep a small "oil bar" in your home:

1. **Collect Basics:** Have castor oil, coconut oil, olive oil, almond oil, and a few essential oils you like.
2. **Designate Tools:** Keep small measuring spoons or droppers, plus a few empty bottles.
3. **Note Results:** Each time you make a mix, record the date, ratio, and any add-ons. Write down how you felt about the smell and texture. This helps you perfect your formulas over time.

This small "lab" approach can be fun and helps you avoid guesswork. Over time, you will learn which blends suit your hair, skin, or personal taste best.

---

## 16. Safety with Essential Oils in Castor Oil

Essential oils are not all the same. Some are safer for skin application, while others can be too harsh. For example, oregano or cinnamon oils can be very strong. If you want to experiment with less common oils, read up on each one's safety guidelines:

- **Check Maximum Dilution:** Some essential oils can only be used at 0.5% to 1% dilution on the skin. That means 1-2 drops in a tablespoon might already be the upper limit.
- **Avoid Certain Oils in Pregnancy:** Some essential oils are not recommended during pregnancy.
- **Keep Out of Eyes and Mouth:** Even if it is in a blend, do not let essential oils near your eyes or mucous membranes.

---

## 17. Using Vinegar or Aloe with Castor Oil?

Some wonder if they can add apple cider vinegar or aloe vera gel to castor oil blends. It is tricky, because vinegar is water-based and does not mix easily with oil. Aloe vera gel also contains water. You would need an emulsifier (a substance that helps oil and water combine) to get a stable mixture. Without it, the product might separate quickly. Some people simply apply aloe or vinegar in a separate step rather than blending them all together in one container.

---

## 18. Specific Goals: Thick Hair vs. Softer Skin

- **Hair Thickening Appearance:** Some folks mix castor oil with Jamaican black castor oil and a bit of rosemary essential oil. They believe it helps the look of fuller hair. Even though strong evidence is still limited, many share positive feedback.
- **Softer Skin:** A combination of castor oil and jojoba oil (equal parts) can act as a quick body moisturizer. Add a drop of lavender if you want a mild smell. Apply right after a shower on slightly damp skin.

---

## 19. Seasonal Adjustments

You might change your blends based on the season:

- **Winter Dryness:** Increase castor oil a bit, or add in thicker oils like shea butter or cocoa butter (melted and mixed in).

- **Summer Heat:** Go with lighter oils like grape seed or fractionated coconut oil. Possibly reduce castor oil to keep it from feeling too heavy on sweaty skin.
- **Humidity:** If you live in a humid place, you might not need as much moisture, so your ratio of castor oil can be smaller.

Keeping track of how your skin and hair react to weather changes can guide you in choosing your blend.

---

## 20. Patch Testing Your Final Blend

You might have tested castor oil alone, but if you add multiple ingredients, you should test the final product again. Dab a small amount on the inside of your forearm or behind your ear. Wait a day. If there is no rash or discomfort, you can move forward. If you notice any reaction, remove it with mild soap and water. Try adjusting your ratio or skipping the ingredient that might be causing trouble.

---

## 21. Selling or Sharing Your Mixes?

Some people enjoy making enough blend to share with friends or family. If you do so:

- **Label It Clearly:** Put all ingredients on the label, plus the date of creation.
- **Warn About Allergens:** If your blend includes common allergens like nut oils, let people know.
- **Legal Rules:** If you plan to sell these blends, there may be local rules about cosmetics manufacturing, labeling, and safety. Do your research to avoid problems.

---

## 22. Building a Routine with Blended Oils

If you have a favorite blend, how do you fit it into daily or weekly life?

- **Morning:** A quick dab for hands or face before stepping out.
- **After Shower:** A body rub while your skin is still damp.
- **Before Bed:** A relaxing scalp or foot massage with a soothing blend.
- **Weekly Hair Mask:** Apply a heavier blend on your scalp or hair, wrap in a towel, wait 20-30 minutes, then wash thoroughly.

By making it a habit, you can see if the mixture is really helping you over time.

---

## 23. Learning from Mistakes

It is easy to make a batch that is too greasy, smells odd, or separates. That is part of the learning process. If a blend is too heavy, add a lighter oil next time. If you do not like the scent, reduce or change the essential oils. If your scalp feels irritated, cut back on stronger oils like peppermint. Keep track of changes in a small notebook or on a phone note app. Over time, you will refine your personal "recipes."

---

## 24. Long-Term Storage Considerations

Some blends might last 6-12 months if all ingredients are stable. However, if you use oils prone to rancidity or if your herbs were not fully dried, the shelf life may be shorter. Signs that your blend is going bad include:

- **Sour or Sharp Smell:** Different from the original scent.
- **Cloudiness or Mold:** Especially in herb-infused oils if moisture was present.
- **Strange Color:** Some natural color changes can happen with herbs, but if it looks off to you, discard it.

When in doubt, make smaller batches so you use them up before they spoil.

# CHAPTER 18: MODERN RESEARCH AND STUDIES

For a long time, castor oil has been part of folk traditions, passed down through families for mild support of the skin, hair, or digestion. Now, as science continues to explore natural products, more researchers are looking at castor oil in controlled settings. In this chapter, we will explore recent findings, the possible reasons behind castor oil's effects, and what still remains to be proven. While not all studies come to the same conclusion, this chapter should give you a sense of how the scientific world sees castor oil today—both the good and the unanswered questions.

## 1. Overview of Scientific Interest in Castor Oil

Research on castor oil dates back many decades, but much of the early work was about its industrial uses (like making plastics or lubricants). Over time, medical and cosmetic researchers also grew curious. They wanted to see if castor oil's unique fatty acid structure—especially ricinoleic acid—gave it special properties. Scientists studied how castor oil might:

- **Influence the skin barrier**
- **Work as a mild laxative**
- **Affect certain germs or fungi**
- **Support general comfort through topical application**

Today, you can find articles in scientific journals looking at castor oil's chemical makeup, its possible activity on the skin, and its effects on lab-grown cells. While not all findings lead to big headlines, they piece together a picture of how castor oil interacts with living tissues.

## 2. Key Role of Ricinoleic Acid

Ricinoleic acid is the main fatty acid in castor oil, making up around 80-90% of its total fatty acids. This is rare among plant oils, as most contain a mix of oleic, linoleic, or other acids. Ricinoleic acid has a hydroxyl group (an -OH part) in its chain, giving it different traits than more common fatty acids. Lab studies have looked at how this might:

- **Change the way cells handle water**
- **Soothe mild swelling**
- **Encourage muscle contractions in the intestines** (which explains the laxative effect)

Some animal tests suggest that ricinoleic acid can affect certain pathways linked to redness or puffiness in tissues. This might be one reason castor oil packs can feel soothing on sore spots. However, more human-based data is needed to confirm these findings widely.

---

## 3. Research on Skin and Wound Care

A few smaller studies have examined castor oil's use in skin ointments or for wound dressing:

- **Moisturizing Effect:** One line of investigation is whether castor oil can help keep skin from losing water. Some trials note that castor oil forms an occlusive layer, reducing water loss. This matches everyday experiences of people using castor oil for dry patches.
- **Wound Healing:** Some hospitals or clinics have tested castor oil-based ointments on bedsores (pressure ulcers) or other small wounds. The thick nature of the oil might help keep the area moist. Reports vary, with some showing positive results and others not seeing a major advantage over standard wound care.
- **Minor Skin Infections:** Because ricinoleic acid has shown some activity against certain germs in lab dishes, there is interest in whether it might help keep small scratches cleaner. Larger or serious infections still require standard medical treatment.

These studies are often small-scale. Larger, more controlled trials would help confirm whether castor oil truly adds value to wound care beyond providing a protective layer.

## 4. Hair Growth Claims Under the Microscope

One of the most popular uses among consumers is castor oil for hair thickness or growth. While there is a large volume of personal stories praising it, formal clinical trials are limited. A few scientific papers note that improved scalp health might reduce breakage, giving the appearance of thicker hair over time. Ricinoleic acid also has mild anti-bacterial or anti-fungal properties, which could keep the scalp cleaner. However, so far there is no large, controlled study proving that castor oil directly speeds up hair growth beyond these indirect improvements.

Still, many individuals remain convinced that regular castor oil applications help them have fuller-looking hair. Researchers say that the "protective coating" and reduced dryness could be the real reason hair appears healthier.

## 5. The Laxative Effect in Clinical Settings

Castor oil has a well-known role as a stimulant laxative. Some older medical texts recommend it for short-term constipation relief. Modern medicine, however, has shifted toward gentler laxatives in many cases, because castor oil can cause strong cramping or diarrhea if overused. Still, there have been small studies:

- **Pregnancy Trials:** A few controlled settings looked at whether castor oil can prompt labor, but results are mixed. Some pregnant people had more frequent contractions, while others just experienced stomach upset.
- **Surgical Prep:** Historically, doctors sometimes used castor oil to clear the intestines before operations. It is less common now, given other bowel-cleansing solutions.

Overall, the scientific consensus is that while castor oil is indeed effective at triggering bowel movements, it should be used sparingly and with caution, especially for those with sensitive systems.

---

## 6. Possible Anti-Inflammatory Actions

As mentioned earlier, some lab experiments suggest that ricinoleic acid might affect pathways involved in swelling. Specifically, it may reduce certain molecules that lead to redness or puffiness. This has led to speculation about castor oil's potential in mild joint or muscle comfort, which is why castor oil packs are used on sore knees or tight muscles. However, large human trials are scarce. Most evidence is either from test tubes or small volunteer studies. If future research confirms these actions in bigger groups, castor oil might gain a more recognized place in certain mild pain management routines.

---

## 7. Studies on Germ and Fungal Control

A handful of experiments have tested castor oil against certain bacteria and fungi:

- **Bacteria:** Some results show that castor oil can reduce the growth of certain Gram-positive bacteria in lab dishes. But real-world use on severe infections is not established.
- **Fungi:** Castor oil might deter some types of fungus that affect the skin or scalp. This could partly explain why some see improvement in dandruff or minor scalp dryness after using castor oil.

Still, these are lab-based findings. Actual infections on human skin are more complicated, and most health workers say standard treatments remain the main approach.

# 8. Research on Castor Oil in Industrial and Cosmetic Production

The cosmetic industry has a separate interest in castor oil. Because it is stable and thick, it is often included in lotions, creams, and lipsticks. It helps achieve certain textures and might prolong the shelf life of some products. Scientists working in product development test how castor oil interacts with other ingredients, ensuring stability. Though this is not purely medical, it influences the variety of consumer products featuring castor oil on the market.

In industrial research, engineers look for ways to use castor oil in biodegradable plastics or lubricants. This side of castor oil research is robust. Many papers detail ways to modify castor oil chemically to create new materials. It goes beyond the scope of personal health but shows how versatile the oil is.

---

# 9. Ongoing Trials and Future Directions

To find out what new research is coming, you can check clinical trial databases or scientific journals. Some areas that may expand in the future:

- **Skin Barrier Research:** Deeper exploration of how castor oil interacts with the outer layer of skin cells.
- **Anti-Inflammatory Pathways:** More rigorous trials to see if castor oil can help mild arthritis or muscle soreness in a measurable way.
- **Topical Delivery of Medicines:** Because castor oil can penetrate the skin to some degree, researchers might see if it can carry certain drugs deeper into tissues.
- **Combining with Modern Ingredients:** Trials that mix castor oil with newer cosmetic molecules to see if they improve product performance.

For the average user, it is helpful to keep an eye on published summaries or reputable health websites that discuss new findings.

## 10. Limitations and Critiques

Critics of castor oil's health uses often point to a lack of large-scale, randomized controlled trials. Many existing studies are small, short, or done on animals or cells in a lab. Also, some older papers are not as rigorously designed as current scientific standards would require. This does not mean castor oil lacks value, but rather that more modern, well-controlled human trials are needed to confirm long-held beliefs. Another critique is that many conclusions are drawn from personal stories rather than data. While personal stories can inspire formal studies, they do not replace systematic research.

---

## 11. Summarizing Known Effects

From the studies so far, we can cautiously say:

1. **Castor Oil as a Laxative:** Well-documented, though it can be harsh, so it should be used with care.
2. **Skin Moisturizing and Protective Layer:** Strong possibility, backed by smaller trials and user reports.
3. **Hair and Scalp Support:** Likely helps by reducing dryness and possibly controlling mild scalp issues, but not proven to regrow hair in a direct sense.
4. **Mild Anti-Inflammatory Activity:** Suggested by lab tests, though larger clinical work is still needed.
5. **Anti-Microbial Aspects:** Shown in test tubes, but real-world evidence is limited to mild or surface-level benefits.

---

## 12. Exploring Ricinoleic Acid in Depth

Because ricinoleic acid is special to castor oil, some labs try to isolate and modify it. They look at how the -OH group can be changed chemically to produce new substances. In a medical sense, the real question is whether ricinoleic acid can be developed into a more targeted medication for swelling or pain. If so, we might see pharmaceutical versions one day. But this is still an emerging area.

## 13. Digital Trends and Anecdotes

In today's digital world, social media platforms and blogs share many personal experiences or "before and after" photos related to castor oil. Researchers sometimes analyze these user posts for patterns. They might see frequent mentions of improved hair look or softer skin after consistent use. While such posts can be biased or unverified, they may lead scientists to form hypotheses about how castor oil might help certain cosmetic goals. Some researchers might then design small trials to test these claims in a more structured way.

## 14. The Role of Large Health Agencies

Major health agencies typically mention castor oil in the context of occasional constipation relief or cosmetic use. They emphasize caution with dosage and remind users about potential side effects. For example, a country's food and drug authority might list castor oil as safe for over-the-counter laxative use if guidelines are followed. However, they rarely endorse it for unproven claims like "cures for major diseases." This measured stance aligns with the fact that most large-scale studies remain to be done.

## 15. Working with Health Professionals

If you are curious about scientific backing and how it might inform your personal use, consider talking with a professional (like a dermatologist for skin concerns or a trichologist for scalp issues). They may have access to the latest research or can interpret studies for your situation. For example, if you want to use castor oil for a scalp condition, they might point you toward a gentle approach or suggest a specific formula. If you have a unique medical condition, a doctor can tell you whether castor oil is compatible with your care plan.

## 16. Research Gaps

- **Long-Term Safety:** We know occasional use is generally safe, but what about daily high use over many years? Studies are limited.
- **Specific Skin Conditions:** Larger trials on eczema, psoriasis, or fungal problems might clarify if castor oil truly helps or if standard treatments are better.
- **Exact Mechanisms of Anti-Inflammatory Activity:** Lab evidence is promising, but we still need well-designed human trials to confirm the best methods, dosages, or frequencies for castor oil packs.
- **Varied Populations:** Studies often focus on small or uniform groups. We need more diverse samples (in terms of age, ethnicity, health background) to see how well results apply to everyone.

## 17. Real-World Examples from Clinics

A few clinics integrate castor oil packs into complementary health programs. They might use them alongside massage or mild exercise for clients with mild joint discomfort. These clinics sometimes keep informal records of how many clients report feeling better. While not as controlled as a formal trial, these "case series" can add to the anecdotal pool. If the results are positive and consistent, it might encourage a researcher to set up a more rigorous study to verify them.

## 18. Balancing Tradition and Science

There is a balance between respecting traditional knowledge—where castor oil has been used for centuries—and applying modern scientific methods to confirm or clarify it. Many natural therapies go through this journey: they start as folk practices, get more attention, and eventually, some become mainstream if evidence supports them. Castor oil is partway through this process. It has mainstream recognition for certain uses (like a laxative or cosmetic ingredient) but remains in the realm of home remedy for others (like hair thickening or certain pack applications).

## 19. The Future of Castor Oil in Health

Looking ahead, we might see:

1. **Improved Formulations:** Scientists could develop castor oil-based creams that target specific conditions, with consistent results.
2. **Medicinal Applications:** If research confirms significant anti-inflammatory effects, a specialized castor oil product might appear on the market for mild joint or muscle complaints.
3. **Regulations and Standards:** Organizations may set stricter standards for labeling castor oil products (e.g., "food-grade," "cosmetic-grade," "therapeutic-grade") to help consumers pick safe and suitable options.
4. **Advanced Studies on Ricinoleic Acid Derivatives:** Chemists might create new compounds from ricinoleic acid that have improved qualities or fewer side effects.

## 20. Impact of Technology on Research

Modern technology lets scientists look deeper into molecular mechanisms. For instance, using advanced imaging, they can see how castor oil layers itself on skin or hair. Tools like electron microscopy or spectrometry help them analyze changes in hair shaft structure after repeated castor oil treatments. We might also see more data-driven approaches, where large sets of user feedback are collected online and analyzed with artificial intelligence to spot patterns. This can guide lab or clinical experiments.

## 21. Gathering Reliable Information

If you want to stay updated:

- **Check Academic Databases:** Online resources like PubMed let you search for "castor oil" and see recent journal articles.
- **Look for Review Articles:** These papers summarize multiple studies, giving a balanced view.
- **Professional Associations:** Groups of dermatologists or pharmacists might publish guidelines.
- **Be Wary of Claims:** Some websites exaggerate castor oil's abilities. Focus on sources that cite actual studies and mention limitations.

---

## 22. Minding Anecdotal vs. Proven

Anecdotal stories can be meaningful, especially when many people report similar experiences, but they are not the same as proven facts. The scientific approach tries to rule out coincidence, placebo effects, and biases. That is why controlled trials are valued. However, in the absence of large trials, many people rely on personal or family experience to decide if castor oil is worth trying. The best path is often a blend of cautious personal testing (like we have described with patch tests and moderate usage) plus staying informed on any new solid data.

---

## 23. Encouraging Collaborative Research

Some observers suggest that universities, natural product companies, and local communities should work together. This can lead to community-based studies where participants use castor oil in a standardized way, track results, and share them with researchers. Such projects might help fill the gap between home use and scientific scrutiny. They could produce medium-sized, real-world data sets that are bigger than individual stories but not as controlled as hospital trials. It is a middle path that might speed up learning about castor oil's real potential.

## 24. Practical Takeaways from Research So Far

- **Use Castor Oil for Mild Support:** The current studies support the idea that it can be a decent choice for occasional dryness, scalp care, or short-term constipation relief.
- **Do Not Over-Rely on It:** Serious skin infections, severe constipation, or big injuries still need professional treatment. Castor oil alone is not enough in those cases.
- **Focus on Quality:** Since some studies point to the importance of pure oil without contaminants, pick a reputable brand.
- **Watch Dosage and Frequency:** Research shows that more is not always better. You want enough to get the effect but not so much that you risk side effects.

# CHAPTER 19: REAL-LIFE STORIES AND HELPFUL EXAMPLES

People often learn best when they see how something works in daily life. Castor oil might sound nice in theory, but it can help to see how real people have used it in simple and practical ways. These stories are not medical advice, but they can show common methods and typical outcomes. In this chapter, we will share a range of examples from different settings—families who have tried castor oil for small concerns, individuals who have worked it into hair routines, and more. By reading their experiences, you might find ideas for your own use. Keep in mind that everyone is different, so you might have different results. Still, these examples can be a helpful guide for those looking to add castor oil into daily tasks.

## 1. A Busy Parent Using Castor Oil Packs for Tired Muscles

A parent named Dana works full-time and cares for three children. She shared that by the end of each day, her lower back and shoulders often felt tight. She read about castor oil packs in an old magazine. One evening, she gave it a try:

- **Preparation:** After dinner, she warmed a bit of castor oil in a small bowl by placing it in warm water. She soaked a soft cloth with the oil.
- **Application:** She rested on her bed, placed the cloth on her lower back, and covered it with plastic wrap and a thin towel. She used a mild heating pad on top.

- **Relaxation Time:** She planned 20 minutes but ended up relaxing for 30 minutes because it felt nice. Her kids watched a show in another room during this time.
- **Results:** Dana reported that her back felt looser afterward, and she enjoyed the short "pause" in her busy routine. She repeated this method a few times each week, saying it helped manage the daily strain.

Dana's story shows how a parent, juggling many tasks, found 20-30 minutes in the evening to apply a castor oil pack for tension. While it did not erase all stress, it gave her a small comfort session. She also warned about the mess factor; the first time she did it, she did not place enough towels underneath and got oil on her sheets. By her second attempt, she laid out old towels and found the process much neater.

---

## 2. College Student's Hair Routine with Castor Oil

Omar, a college student living in a dorm, had always heard that castor oil might help with hair dryness. He tried to grow his hair longer, but it looked dull at the ends. Here is what he did:

- **Mixing a Simple Hair Oil:** Omar blended 1 part castor oil with 1 part coconut oil in a small plastic bottle.
- **Application Before Showering:** Twice a week, he lightly dampened his hair, then rubbed a spoonful of the mix into his scalp and worked the rest through the ends. He put on a shower cap for about 20 minutes while he tidied his room.
- **Washing Out:** When he showered, he used a clarifying shampoo, sometimes rinsing twice to avoid leftover oil. He followed up with a mild conditioner.
- **Observed Changes:** After a month, Omar felt his hair looked shinier and less frizzy. He did not see dramatic growth, but he noticed fewer split ends. The routine also became a small self-care habit.

Omar's example indicates that using a castor oil blend regularly can make hair appear more hydrated. The key step for him was thorough washing, so he did not have an oily scalp. He also realized that for his fine hair, a 1:1 ratio was enough to avoid feeling weighed down.

---

## 3. Mild Constipation Relief for an Older Adult (with Doctor's Advice)

Mr. Chan is in his seventies and sometimes has mild constipation. He heard that older people can be more sensitive to strong laxatives, so he consulted his doctor about castor oil:

- **Doctor's Guidance:** The doctor suggested a small measured amount, specifically around 1 teaspoon if constipation persisted, and advised him not to exceed 1 tablespoon in extreme cases.
- **Usage Method:** Mr. Chan took 1 teaspoon of food-grade castor oil mixed in orange juice in the morning if he had not had a bowel movement in two days.
- **Results and Caution:** He found that within a few hours, it worked well, but he needed to stay near the bathroom. He also had to drink water to avoid feeling weak. His doctor told him not to make this a weekly habit—only once in a while if fiber or other gentle methods failed.

Mr. Chan's story reminds us that castor oil can be potent internally, so older adults must measure carefully and stay hydrated. His approach worked with professional guidance, showing that castor oil can fit into an overall plan but should not be the first or everyday step for chronic issues.

---

## 4. Young Adult Experimenting with Castor Oil for Eyebrows and Lashes

Many online posts talk about castor oil for thicker eyebrows or eyelashes. Maria, a 25-year-old, decided to try it. She bought a clean mascara wand and did the following:

- **Nightly Routine:** After washing her face, she dipped the wand in castor oil (making sure it was not dripping) and lightly brushed her brows. Then, very carefully, she brushed her lashes, avoiding the eye area.
- **Outcome Over Weeks:** For the first week, she noticed no change. By the second month, she felt her brows looked a bit fuller. However, she was not sure if it was new growth or just less breakage. Her eyelashes also felt stronger, but not significantly longer.
- **Pros and Cons:** She liked that the oil was cheap and easy, but disliked that she had to be careful not to get it in her eyes. She sometimes found it sticky if she used too much.

Maria concluded that while castor oil might not magically transform lashes, it can help them look healthy by reducing dryness. She also warned friends to do a patch test and to keep the oil away from direct contact with eyes.

---

## 5. Small-Scale Home Project: Lip Balm for the Whole Family

In one family, two teens and their mother decided to make homemade lip balms for fun. They used a simple recipe with castor oil, beeswax, and a drop of peppermint essential oil:

- **Process:** They melted 1 tablespoon of beeswax pellets, then stirred in 1 tablespoon of castor oil and 1 tablespoon of coconut oil. After taking it off the heat, they added 1 drop of peppermint oil.
- **Pouring and Cooling:** They poured the mix into small tin containers. Once cooled, the balm hardened.
- **Family Feedback:** Each person tested it. They found it thicker than store-bought chapstick, but it gave a nice protective layer on the lips. The slight peppermint flavor was pleasant, though the father found it a bit tingly.
- **Shelf Life:** They stored extra tins in a drawer. After about three months, the leftover tins still smelled normal. The mother reminded everyone not to expose them to direct sun or leave them in a hot car.

This example shows a family activity that introduced castor oil in a creative way. It also taught the teens basic steps of measuring and melting. The mother made sure they used minimal essential oil to avoid irritation.

---

## 6. A Runner's Experience with Castor Oil on Feet

Trina runs multiple times a week. Her feet often develop calluses and dryness around the heels. She tried many lotions but decided to give castor oil a try, especially after reading about foot soaks:

- **Routine:** Once a week, Trina soaked her feet in warm water with a pinch of Epsom salt for about 10 minutes. Then she dried them well.
- **Applying Oil:** She massaged a teaspoon of castor oil into each foot, focusing on the heel and any callused parts. She put on loose cotton socks and relaxed for 15 minutes, reading a book.
- **Outcome:** She noted that after a month, her heels were less rough, though not perfectly smooth. She continued this method, cutting back on it in the summer months when her schedule changed.
- **Tips:** Trina recommended wearing socks to avoid slipping around the house. She also trimmed thick calluses gently before applying oil to let it soak in better.

Trina's story is a direct example of how castor oil can help dryness in feet. The soak plus oil approach gave her a small weekly foot care ritual that made running more comfortable.

---

## 7. Young Couple's Try with Castor Oil for Mild Tummy Aches

James and Lena occasionally have mild tummy aches due to either stress or certain foods. They read about castor oil packs for the abdomen:

- **Method:** They folded a small cloth, soaked it in castor oil, and placed it on the lower abdomen. They did not use heat at first, just the oil and a layer of plastic wrap. They lay still for 20 minutes.

- **Results:** James reported feeling a bit calmer afterward. Lena sometimes used a warm towel on top, saying it felt more soothing. They found it worked best for mild bloating, but not for stronger pains. If they had ongoing discomfort, they would look into diet changes or talk to a health worker.
- **Cautions:** They noticed that the cloth could stain clothes if they were not careful. So they made dedicated "castor oil pack towels."

Their shared experience underlines that a castor oil pack can be a small comfort measure. It is not a replacement for real medical care, but for everyday mild issues, it can be part of an overall plan.

---

## 8. A High School Teacher Using Castor Oil for Hand Care

Mrs. Patel, a high school teacher, washes her hands frequently, especially during cold and flu season. She found her hands became chapped and dry:

- **Evening Hand Rub:** She began keeping a small bottle of castor oil mixed with olive oil (about 1:2 ratio) near her sink. After her evening wash, she patted her hands dry and rubbed a few drops of the oil blend into her palms and cuticles.
- **Results Over Time:** By the end of a month, she noticed fewer cracks on her knuckles. She also found that her cuticles looked softer, making it easier to keep her nails neat.
- **Additional Tips:** She sometimes wore thin cotton gloves if the dryness was severe, but usually did not need to. She advised her fellow teachers to try a similar blend, though some did not like the smell of olive oil.

This example shows that a quick rub with a castor-based blend can help those who wash their hands often. It is simple, does not require heating or packs, and fits into a daily routine.

---

## 9. Grandparent's View of Using Castor Oil in Past Times

Mr. Ruiz, in his late eighties, recalls that his mother used castor oil for many small problems:

- **Historic Use:** He remembered her giving him a spoonful when he was "backed up," and also using it on minor scrapes. At times, he found it unpleasant to swallow, but it did clear him out quickly.
- **Changes Over Time:** Mr. Ruiz notes that modern families have more options (fiber supplements, gentle creams, etc.), so castor oil is not as commonly forced on kids as in his youth. But he still feels it has a place, especially in small amounts for dryness or an occasional pack.
- **Message to Younger Folks:** He warns not to assume castor oil is a miracle for all ills, but also not to dismiss it. He says that with the right knowledge, it is a decent item to keep in a household kit.

This glimpse into older practices shows how castor oil was once a go-to solution. While times have changed, the underlying principle—use it wisely—remains.

---

## 10. Friend Group Testing a Homemade Soap with Castor Oil

A group of friends decided to attempt cold-process soap making, using an online recipe that included castor oil:

- **Recipe Basics:** The recipe called for olive oil, coconut oil, castor oil, and lye in specific amounts. Castor oil was about 5-10% of the total.
- **Production:** They followed safety steps with lye, blending the oils until "trace" formed. After pouring into molds, they let it cure for several weeks.
- **Finished Soap:** The bar had a nice lather and felt slightly more moisturizing than a plain coconut/olive soap. They all liked how their hands felt after washing.
- **Lessons:** They learned that castor oil helps create a stable, creamy foam in handmade soap. They also realized that exact

measurements are crucial. One friend used too much castor oil in a small batch, leading to a softer bar that took longer to harden.

This example is more advanced, but it shows another angle of castor oil use: soap making. The group discovered that castor oil can improve the lather's quality, which is why many DIY soap enthusiasts include it in recipes.

---

## 11. Athlete Using Castor Oil for Sore Knees

Carlos, a basketball player in his twenties, had mild knee discomfort after intense games. He wanted a natural approach to go along with his stretching routine:

- **Creating a Simple Rub**: He mixed 1 tablespoon castor oil with 1 tablespoon of grapeseed oil and 2 drops of rosemary essential oil.
- **Application**: After practice, he iced his knees briefly, then did a light rub with the oil mixture. He did not do a full pack, just a short massage.
- **Feeling Over Time**: He said he found the mild warmth from the oil rub comforting, though it was not a cure. Combined with rest and elevation, his knees felt less tight.
- **Advice to Others**: He suggested that players check with a sports doctor if they have serious issues. For him, it was more of a small measure to calm muscle tension around the knee.

This story highlights that castor oil rubs can be part of a post-exercise routine. However, it is just one piece of muscle and joint care, alongside icing, stretching, and rest.

---

## 12. Bakery Owner Using Castor Oil on Dry Elbows

Michelle runs a bakery, spending long hours mixing dough and washing pans. The constant contact with flour and water left her elbows rough and flaky:

- **Evening Lotion:** She poured 2 tablespoons of castor oil and 2 tablespoons of almond oil into a small pump bottle, shaking it before each use.
- **Quick Application:** Each night, she pumped a small amount onto her elbows and rubbed gently. If she had extra, she rubbed it on her arms.
- **Outcome:** Within a couple of weeks, the dryness improved. She still needed to exfoliate the elbows in the shower sometimes, but the oil blend kept the skin from cracking.
- **Note on Smell:** Michelle added a tiny drop of vanilla extract (food-grade) to give the blend a mild sweet smell. She said it was optional but made it more pleasant.

Michelle's example is straightforward: a simple daily rub can help dryness caused by repeated washing. She found that a balanced blend of castor oil with a lighter oil made it easier to handle.

---

## 13. Teen's Cautionary Tale of Overusing Castor Oil on Face

Tony, 16, read that castor oil could help clear blemishes. He applied pure castor oil nightly, hoping to reduce spots:

- **Problem:** After a week, his pores felt clogged, and he developed more bumps on his forehead. His parents took him to a doctor, who explained that castor oil can be heavy for some teens prone to breakouts.
- **Solution:** The doctor suggested a milder face cleanser and told him to stop using heavy oils on his face. Over time, Tony's skin improved once he switched to lighter, non-comedogenic products.
- **Tony's Lesson:** He realized that not all natural products are good for every person, especially if they have specific skin issues like acne.

This cautionary tale shows that while castor oil helps dryness, it can be too thick for some facial skin types, leading to clogging. Always consider your own skin type or get advice if unsure.

## 14. Friends Trying Castor Oil for Dandruff

Two friends, Dan and Felix, both had mild flakes on their scalp. They decided to try a castor oil scalp mask:

- **Preparation:** They mixed castor oil with a bit of jojoba oil and a few drops of tea tree essential oil (since it is known for scalp concerns).
- **Application:** They each massaged the blend into the scalp, focusing on flaky zones, and left it for 15-20 minutes before shampooing thoroughly.
- **Results:** Dan noticed fewer flakes after a few sessions, while Felix did not see much change. They guessed that Felix's flakes might be linked to something else (maybe dryness from certain hair products), so he decided to see a dermatologist.
- **Observation:** Dan was convinced that the mild anti-fungal aspect of tea tree plus castor oil's moisturizing effect helped him. Felix concluded he needed a different approach.

This pair example shows that what works for one person may not work for another. Dandruff can have varied causes, and castor oil plus tea tree might help if it is mild dryness or mild scalp issues, but not if it is a more persistent condition.

## 15. A Short Story of Castor Oil in Pets (External Use Only)

An owner named Lee had a dog with rough paw pads:

- **Method:** Lee dabbed a tiny bit of castor oil on a cotton ball and patted it onto the dog's paw pads after a walk. Then wiped off any excess with a tissue so the dog would not slip on the floor.
- **Result:** The paw pads seemed less cracked. The dog did not mind the routine, and after a couple of weeks, the dryness eased.
- **Vet's Input:** The veterinarian reminded Lee to use a small amount and prevent the dog from licking it too much. It was safe in small external amounts, but not recommended for internal use or large areas.

Though we covered pet caution in an earlier chapter, this short story shows a real-life example of using castor oil safely on a dog's paws to relieve dryness.

---

## 16. A Mentor Teaching Teenagers Soap Making with Castor Oil

Ms. Lane runs a community workshop for teens. She introduced them to beginner soap making:

- **Plan:** She provided materials for a simple cold-process recipe that used coconut oil, olive oil, and 5% castor oil. She showed them how to handle lye safely, measure oils, and mix everything.
- **Outcome:** Each teen got to pour soap into small molds. After a few weeks of curing, they tested the bars at home.
- **Feedback:** The teens liked the creamy foam. Some gave bars to family as gifts. Ms. Lane told them about castor oil's thick nature and how it can boost lather in homemade soap. They learned not to use too much, or the soap can become soft or sticky.

This shows how castor oil is relevant not just in personal care but also as part of educational craft projects that teach chemistry, safety, and creativity.

---

## 17. Group of Friends Doing a "Castor Oil Spa Night"

Three friends, each dealing with mild dryness in different places, planned a home spa night:

- **Facial Steam and Light Mask:** One friend used a small dab of castor oil on her forehead after steaming. She kept it on for 10 minutes, then rinsed it off.
- **Foot Soak:** Another friend soaked feet in warm water, then applied castor oil, wearing socks for half an hour.

- **Scalp Massage:** The third friend parted her hair in sections, massaging castor oil and a dash of coconut oil at the roots.
- **Shared Observations:** They played calming music, chatted, and found the process relaxing. By the end of the night, each reported smoother skin or scalp. They also noted the mess factor, so they spread old towels on the floor.

This group experience demonstrates how castor oil can bring people together in a small, low-cost spa setup. Each person chose a method that fit their own dryness issues, turning it into a casual, supportive evening.

## 18. Real-Life Steps to Avoid Overuse

A young adult, Elijah, found that castor oil helped his scalp dryness. He got excited and began applying it daily. Soon, his hair felt heavy, and he had to shampoo multiple times to remove buildup. Eventually, he limited the scalp oiling to once or twice a week:

- **Adjusting Frequency:** He saw that daily use was unnecessary and that less frequent but consistent sessions were more effective.
- **Better Balance:** After the change, his scalp stayed comfortable, and he did not spend forever washing his hair. He learned that more product was not always better.

This reminds us that using castor oil in moderation can be more efficient than daily, heavy application, especially for the hair or scalp.

## 19. Observing Changes During Seasons

Sarah lived in a place with cold winters and humid summers. She used castor oil-based lotions in winter but switched to a lighter approach in summer:

- **Winter Mode:** She added extra castor oil to her usual lotion, about 1:1, to help keep skin from drying out in heated indoor air.

- **Summer Mode:** She cut castor oil to about 1:3 with a lighter oil (like grapeseed oil). She also used less product overall due to sweat and higher humidity.
- **Result:** Sarah found that adjusting the ratio by season gave her consistent comfort without feeling too greasy.

Her approach shows how environment can affect castor oil routines. She used different blends for different seasons, making sure her skin stayed balanced.

---

## 20. Final Thoughts on Everyday Uses

All these real-life stories share a few common points. First, castor oil is versatile, but each person must adapt it to their own needs. Second, small details matter—like measuring, picking the right ratio, or leaving enough time for clean-up. Third, results can vary a lot. One person's success might not be yours, especially if your body or hair type is different. Fourth, mixing castor oil with other oils or mild ingredients is often helpful for texture and effect.

The main lesson is that castor oil can be a simple item that many people include in small personal routines. It does not require fancy equipment—just some knowledge of how to apply it, how to store it, and how often to use it. These stories do not replace medical insight, but they can spark ideas and show how castor oil fits into real homes, from busy parents to craft-loving teens. As we move on, we will wrap up the final chapter with a list of common questions and some parting thoughts. By now, you should have plenty of insights into how castor oil can become a practical helper in daily life.

---

# CHAPTER 20: COMMON QUESTIONS AND FINAL THOUGHTS

After going through many chapters about castor oil—its background, ways to use it, safety, and stories from everyday experiences—you might still have some questions. This closing chapter will address many of the typical ones that come up. It will also offer final thoughts on how to decide if castor oil is right for you and how to keep learning more about its potential. Castor oil is neither a cure for every problem nor something to dismiss. Used carefully, it can be part of a practical routine for mild concerns. Let's look at the frequently asked questions and wrap up our entire discussion in a clear manner.

## 1. Is Castor Oil Safe for Everyone?

Many people can use castor oil safely, but there are exceptions:

- **Allergies or Skin Sensitivities**: Some people develop redness or itching. A patch test can help you find out if you are sensitive.
- **Health Conditions**: If you have a serious condition, especially linked to digestion or skin, ask a health professional before using castor oil (internally or externally).
- **Pregnant Individuals**: Swallowing castor oil can cause strong bowel movements that may stress the body. Seek professional advice if considering it during pregnancy.
- **Children**: Be extra cautious with internal use. External uses like a short foot rub may be fine, but keep an eye on them.

In short, castor oil is generally recognized as safe in moderate amounts, but personal factors matter.

## 2. Which Type of Castor Oil Should I Buy?

Look for labels that meet your intended use:

- **Food-Grade or Laxative Label:** If you plan on swallowing it for occasional constipation, be sure it says "food-grade" or has instructions for that purpose.
- **Cosmetic or Skin Use:** A bottle might say "cold-pressed" or "pure." Jamaican black castor oil is a variant some prefer for hair but can be heavier in color and smell.
- **Organic Options:** Some users choose organic to ensure fewer chemicals were used in the growing process, though it might cost more.

## 3. How Do I Store Castor Oil Properly?

Place the bottle in a cool, dark spot. Some keep it in a cupboard or closet, away from direct sun or heat. Ensure the cap is sealed tightly. If you see changes in color or smell, it may be old. Replace if it smells rancid or strange. Most castor oil lasts at least a year or more when stored well.

## 4. How Often Can I Use a Castor Oil Pack?

This depends on what you are targeting. Some people do it once or twice a week for mild issues. Others might do it daily for a short period, but that can be messy or time-consuming. Pay attention to your skin's reaction. If you see dryness or any signs of irritation, reduce the frequency. Castor oil packs are typically not meant for daily, lifelong use—more as an occasional supportive measure.

## 5. Can I Use Castor Oil on My Face if I Get Pimples?

Some users with oily or pimple-prone skin find castor oil too thick. However, others use a light "oil cleansing method" with a small ratio of castor oil mixed with a lighter oil, massaging it gently and rinsing it off. If you try it, do a small test first. If pimples worsen, it might not be suitable for your skin type.

---

## 6. Are There Safe Ways to Put Castor Oil Near the Eyes?

If you want to use it on eyebrows or eyelashes, do so cautiously:

- **Use a Clean Brush or Wand:** And do not overload the brush.
- **Stay Clear of the Eye:** Focus on brow hair or lash tips.
- **Patch Test:** The skin around the eyes can be extra sensitive.
- **Stop if You Feel Irritation:** Rinse with water if it gets into the eye.

---

## 7. Can Castor Oil Really Make Hair Grow Faster?

No large scientific study confirms that castor oil directly boosts the speed of hair growth. It may help hair look fuller by reducing dryness or breakage, and some people anecdotally report seeing improvements. But as of now, there is no solid proof that it changes the rate at which hair grows from the follicles. It is more likely helping hair stay healthier so it can reach its potential length without as much breakage.

---

## 8. What If I Have a Reaction?

If you notice redness, itching, or a rash, wash the area with mild soap and water. You can also apply a gentle moisturizer without castor oil. If symptoms persist or worsen, seek medical guidance. Reactions are rare but can happen, as with any product.

## 9. How Much Castor Oil Is Too Much When Swallowed?

It depends on the person's size, age, and health. Generally, 1 teaspoon to 1 tablespoon is a typical adult dose for occasional constipation. More than that may cause severe cramps or diarrhea. If you accidentally take too much, drink water, and watch for signs of dehydration. If you are worried, call a health professional. Regular large doses can lead to problems, so it is not recommended.

## 10. Do I Need to Warm the Oil for External Use?

Warming can help the oil spread better and feel nicer, but it is not always mandatory. Some people apply it at room temperature. If you do warm it, do not make it too hot—just warm enough so it is comfortable. You can place a small bowl of castor oil in a larger bowl of warm water for a few minutes.

## 11. Is Jamaican Black Castor Oil Better?

"Better" is subjective. Jamaican black castor oil is made by roasting the seeds, which changes color, smell, and possibly some minor qualities. Some people swear by it for hair, but others find the smell too strong or the consistency too thick. It is a personal choice. Both regular castor oil and Jamaican black castor oil contain ricinoleic acid. The difference often lies in color, smell, and small changes in pH or ash content from roasting.

## 12. Can I Use Castor Oil in the Kitchen for Cooking?

Typically, people do not use castor oil as a cooking oil because it has a strong taste and a known laxative effect. Even though it is derived from a plant seed, it is not commonly chosen for frying or baking. If you see castor oil labeled "food-grade," that primarily means it is safe for occasional oral use, not that it is a typical cooking product.

## 13. Why Does Castor Oil Smell or Taste Strong?

Castor oil has a distinct aroma, sometimes described as earthy or slightly pungent. Jamaican black castor oil can smell stronger due to the roasting process. The taste is often disliked because it is quite thick, with a lingering aftertaste. That is why people who swallow it mix it with juice or something else to mask the flavor.

## 14. What If My Castor Oil Gets Cloudy?

Some oils change consistency if stored in cooler places, leading to a cloudy look. This does not always mean it is spoiled. Warm it gently and see if it clears up. Check the scent—if it smells sour, that is a hint it might be going bad. If it still smells normal and the cloudiness disappears upon warming, it is likely okay to use.

## 15. Can I Freeze Castor Oil?

There is not much need to freeze it. It usually stays fine in a cool cupboard for a decent time. Freezing might change its texture or cause partial separation. If you do freeze it, let it thaw at room temperature before use, and shake if needed. Always check for smell or color changes if you stored it in an unusual way.

## 16. Are There Any Great Tools for Applying Castor Oil?

For hair or lashes, some use clean mascara wands, droppers, or small brushes. For skin, you can use your hands, cotton pads, or reusable cloth squares. For scalp areas, some prefer nozzle bottles that let them direct the oil in small lines. None of these are mandatory, but the right tool can reduce mess and make application easier.

## 17. How Do I Choose a Good Brand?

Look for:

- **Clear Labeling:** Does it say how it was pressed (cold-pressed, expeller-pressed)? Does it mention if it is for cosmetic or food use?
- **Reputation:** Check reviews or ask friends. Some widely recognized brands have consistent quality.
- **Packaging:** A seal that shows it was not tampered with. A dark bottle if possible.
- **Certifications:** If you want organic, check for reputable organic seals.

## 18. Can Castor Oil Help With Scars?

Scars are tricky. Some people say castor oil keeps the scar area softer, which might reduce itching or dryness. But thick scars need more specialized treatments. Castor oil alone will not remove deep scarring or fully erase old marks. It might help keep the skin moisturized, which can make scars less noticeable, but results vary greatly.

## 19. How Does Castor Oil Compare to Other Home Remedies?

Each home remedy has its own traits. For instance, coconut oil is lighter and has a mild smell, while olive oil has a more robust scent. Castor oil stands out for its thickness and high ricinoleic acid content. If you want a simpler or thinner oil for daily moisturizing, you might pick a different one.

But if you need a heavier occlusive layer, castor oil might be the best choice. People often keep more than one oil on hand for different tasks.

## 20. What if I See No Improvement?

If you have used castor oil in a certain way (for example, on dry skin or hair dryness) for several weeks and see no change, you might:

- **Adjust the Method:** Try a different ratio or add a gentle exfoliation step.
- **Reduce Frequency:** Daily might be too much, or weekly might be too little. Experiment.
- **Check External Factors:** Diet, stress, or other products might be overshadowing castor oil's effects.
- **Get a Second Opinion:** If the issue is significant, see a dermatologist or other specialist.

Not everyone responds the same. It might help to keep a brief diary of your usage to track changes over time.

## 21. Should I Use Castor Oil Alongside Other Treatments?

If you are already treating a condition—like using medicated creams or prescription laxatives—talk to your health worker before adding castor oil. Some conflicts could arise if it changes how your skin absorbs certain meds, or if taking it internally affects other medications. In many mild cases, it might be fine, but it is always safer to be sure.

## 22. Could Castor Oil Become More Popular Soon?

Interest in natural items has grown. Castor oil, being plant-based and versatile, might continue to be part of that trend. Ongoing research and user stories keep it relevant. As more people share experiences on social media, castor oil gains new fans who try it out of curiosity. It is not likely to vanish from shelves anytime soon. Major personal care brands sometimes add it in formulas, too. So you can expect to see it in stores and online for years to come.

## 23. Final Advice for Beginners

1. **Start Small:** If you are new to castor oil, begin with a small area or a low dose.
2. **Observe Your Body's Response:** Everyone is unique. Watch for dryness, breakouts, or any sign that it is not helping.
3. **Blend If Needed:** If pure castor oil feels too sticky, mix it with a lighter oil.
4. **Stay Patient:** Improvements might take weeks for hair or skin changes. It is not usually a quick fix.
5. **Ask Questions:** If unsure, check with a health worker or look for reliable info online, focusing on sites that refer to actual data.

## 24. Looking Ahead

Castor oil has been in use for centuries, and it is still relevant today. Though some of its claims are not backed by huge trials, many people find real value in it for dryness, mild hair support, or occasional bowel help. Because it is generally affordable and widely available, it remains a first try for many. Future studies might confirm more about its chemical pathways, or new products might come out that harness specific parts of castor oil in refined ways.

Either way, castor oil sits at the intersection of tradition and ongoing exploration. Whether you just keep a small bottle for an occasional pack or integrate it into a weekly hair routine, it can be a supportive item in a balanced personal care plan. Remember to use common sense, watch for any issues, and enjoy the process if it suits you.

# 25. Closing Thoughts on Castor Oil

We have traveled through castor oil's history, chemistry, uses, safety steps, and real-life stories. The main points are:

- **Know What It Is and How It Works:** Ricinoleic acid is key, giving castor oil its thickness and possible soothing effects.
- **Use It Carefully:** Measure doses if swallowing, do patch tests on skin, and follow a sensible routine.
- **Try Blending:** Often, mixing it with other oils or herbs can enhance ease of use and target specific needs.
- **Respect Limits:** For serious issues, see a health professional. Castor oil is a mild helper, not a replacement for medical care.
- **Stay Open to Learning:** Research is ongoing, so keep an eye out for new findings.

Castor oil can be a reliable part of a home kit if you use it with awareness. Its range of applications—from hair to skin and beyond—makes it worth exploring, as long as you remain informed and cautious. We hope this book has given you the knowledge and confidence to use castor oil in simple, practical ways suited to your needs. Whether you do a once-a-week hair mask or an occasional abdominal pack, remember that small changes in your routine can add up to a more comfortable, balanced daily life.

www.ingramcontent.com/pod-product-compliance
Lightning Source LLC
LaVergne TN
LVHW012042070526
838202LV00056B/5569